Unseen

Breda O'Toole is a music teacher, a mother of eight, three of whom died as babies, and a grandmother of twelve. She lives in Connemara, County Galway.

Dr Tony Bates is a clinical psychologist and Adjunct Professor of Psychology at University College Dublin. He was Head of the Department of Psychology for 30 years at St James's Hospital Dublin. Following psychotherapy training at the University of Pennsylvania and the University of Oxford, he established the MSc in Cognitive Psychotherapy at Trinity College Dublin. In 2006, he created Jigsaw (The National Centre for Youth Mental Health). He trained as a mindfulness teacher at the University of North Wales, Bangor, in 2001 and is patron of the Mindfulness Teachers Association of Ireland. Tony lives on a headland in north Sligo.

Unseen

A MEMOIR OF TRAUMA,
IRELAND'S PSYCHIATRIC SYSTEM
AND A LIFETIME SPENT HEALING

Breda O'Toole

with **DR TONY BATES**
and **LIA HYNES**

Gill Books

Gill Books
Hume Avenue
Park West
Dublin 12
www.gillbooks.ie

Gill Books is an imprint of M.H. Gill and Co.

© Breda O'Toole 2025

978 18045 83364

This book does not in any way represent medical advice for individual persons. Readers are advised to attend their own healthcare professionals for advice and guidance appropriate to their particular needs. This book does not in any way replace the advice and guidance that your own doctor or other healthcare professional can give you. If you are concerned about any of the issues raised in this book, be sure to consult your doctor.

Design origination by O'K Graphic Design, Dublin
Edited by Sally Vince
Proofread by Geraldine Begley
Printed and bound in the UK using 100% renewable electricity
at CPI Group (UK) Ltd
This book is typeset in Minion Pro by Palimpsest Book Production Limited, Falkirk, Stirlingshire

The paper used in this book comes from the wood pulp of sustainably managed forests.

All rights reserved.

No part of this publication may be copied, reproduced or transmitted in any form or by any means, without written permission of the publishers.

To the best of our knowledge, this book complies in full with the requirements of the General Product Safety Regulation (GPSR). For further information and help with any safety queries, please contact us at productsafety@gill.ie.

A CIP catalogue record for this book is available from the British Library.

5 4 3 2 1

To my beloved family – Tommy; our children, Dermot, Francis, Peter (in loving memory), Fiona, Karen, Maria, Breda Ann and Marguerite; my sons-in-law; extended family members and relatives; and all my wonderful grandchildren. Each of you holds a special place in my heart that words alone cannot fully express.

This book is also dedicated to those who endure the persistent struggles of trauma, pain, mental anguish and distress in any form. Our shared journey of endurance, resilience and courage binds us together. You are forever in my heart.

CONTENTS

Foreword by Tony Bates   xi

October 1973, St Brigid's Hospital, Ballinasloe   1

Part One: The two arrows

	INTRODUCTION	5
CHAPTER 1	WHERE IT ALL BEGAN	7
CHAPTER 2	GROWING UP IN THE SHADOW OF TRAUMA	14
CHAPTER 3	IN SEARCH OF AN IDENTITY	29
CHAPTER 4	LOOKING FOR ANSWERS	41
CHAPTER 5	FALLING APART	49

Part Two: Unheard

CHAPTER 6	THE PSYCHIATRIST	65
CHAPTER 7	WEDDING DAY BLUES	88
CHAPTER 8	THE NURSE WHO RISKED EVERYTHING	97
CHAPTER 9	THANK YOU FOR HEARING ME	106
CHAPTER 10	A MOTHER KNOWS	111
CHAPTER 11	GIVING SORROW WORDS	117
CHAPTER 12	A CRY OF PAIN	135
CHAPTER 13	FINDING HOPE	153
CHAPTER 14	OVERCOMING VALIUM ADDICTION	166

CHAPTER 15	MY STRUGGLE TO MOTHER	173
CHAPTER 16	MY MOTHER	180
CHAPTER 17	RECLAIMING MY MIND	190
CHAPTER 18	SICK OF BEING SICK	206

Part Three: Loving the stranger who was myself

CHAPTER 19	MY 'ONE GOOD ADULT'	219
CHAPTER 20	LEARNING TO BE A MOTHER	230
CHAPTER 21	CHANGES AND HABITS THAT HELPED	235
CHAPTER 22	WHAT'S GOD GOT TO DO WITH IT?	255
CHAPTER 23	LETTING GO OF RESENTMENT	259
CHAPTER 24	ACCESSING MY MEDICAL FILES	270
CHAPTER 25	WRITING THIS BOOK	280
CHAPTER 26	A PLACE OF BELONGING	289

A LETTER TO PSYCHIATRY: A COMPLAINT AGAINST MY CARE	295
GLOSSARY OF MEDICATIONS AND TREATMENTS ADMINISTERED TO BREDA	299
ACKNOWLEDGEMENTS	301

'We have two lives ... the life we learn with and the life we live after that.'

Bernard Malamud, *The Natural*

FOREWORD

I first met Breda when she approached me at the Clifden Arts Festival to tell me that she found a particular story I had shared with the audience very moving. It was about a profoundly vulnerable young man who had spent most of his life in psychiatric care. A couple of years before he tragically succumbed to cancer, he experienced a remarkable recovery from lifelong episodes of psychosis and lived a full, medication-free life.

Breda connected personally with this story. The cruelty of her early life had left her emotionally scarred. The traumas she bore painfully in her body for years began to catch up with her as a young adult, prompting her to seek help from psychiatry.

The culture of care in psychiatry that Breda turned to was a culture of fear. I was part of our mental health system during the time she engaged with it. We felt afraid of the profound emotional suffering we faced daily in our 'patients', as we feared encountering those same depths within ourselves. We prioritised objectivity and detachment over genuinely engaging with individuals in their pain. We remained spectators of those trapped in the shadows of a tormented inner world.

Some staff, mainly nurses, were unafraid. They had a natural ease born of years of working closely with mental torment. They saw through the noise of 'psychiatric symptoms' to the person behind them. They understood intuitively how much people in pain need to be seen and heard. Only when they felt listened to and accepted could they retrieve their lost sense of dignity. However, wise and compassionate carers were the exception rather than the norm.

Breda was admitted to psychiatric hospitals for over 23 years (1972–95) and received multiple medications that caused debilitating side effects. She was an accomplished musician who had studied under Seán Ó Riada. However, after undergoing 29 electroconvulsive treatments, she lost the memory of all the music she had learned and has since suffered from recurring headaches.

The most painful part of her experiences of psychiatric care was that – with one exception – she remained 'unseen' as a person and her story 'unheard'. No one ever seemed to take the time to understand why an intelligent, loving mother was finding her life impossible.

Breda's experiences of psychiatric care were not merely ineffective; they kept her trapped in repetitive cycles of misery rather than offering any hope of recovery.

By any standard, this was unacceptable. Perhaps one explanation for why her care was so unsuccessful lies in how psychiatry viewed mental ill health at that time. A person's distress was considered the result of a chemical imbalance or brain disease. Family, childhood and social traumas that led to emotional and relational problems were ignored or downplayed. We looked for what was 'wrong' with people instead of asking what had happened to them. A person's sadness, anxiety, rage or profound loneliness was seen as something medically 'wrong' with them that required 'treatment' through medication. Services appeared unable or unwilling to explore alternative explanations.

In the mid-90s, Breda stepped away from psychiatric care, weaned herself off all of her prescribed medications, and, with the help of a therapist, faced key traumas in her life that had never been addressed previously. Her recovery involved many twists and turns, but she ultimately discovered herself to be someone she could believe in and love.

Our recent mental health policies recognise the vital role that childhood trauma, family dysfunction and social disadvantage play in our mental health vulnerabilities. They also emphasise the necessity for each individual to participate in developing a meaningful recovery plan. Medication may assist in stabilising a person to confront painful issues in their lives, but it is never the solution to emotional pain.

Despite these impressive advances, I am concerned that the current emphasis on chasing symptoms and tinkering with medication regimens still blinds us to the human elements involved in emotional distress. Neglecting the significance of human connections for people who already feel isolated and alone leaves them even more demoralised.

Breda's experience shows how harmful it can be to ignore the undertow of unresolved traumas that repeatedly trip people up. By contrast, it also shows how healing it can be to find a skilled therapist and have the support of family and friends to rely on.

Her story is unique because she took pains to track down and collate her medical records from each hospital where she was admitted. Daily nursing notes, medical reports and discharge summaries document how she was viewed and treated.

Breda writes not from a place of anger or as a 'victim', but as someone who has reclaimed her life, transforming her suffering into compassion for those who struggle. Her story will resonate with many, particularly those who have been disabled, rather than enabled, by our mental health services.

This book is a gift from her heart to each of us. Breda's journey out of her darkness, overcoming seemingly insurmountable obstacles, is empowering. Her hard-won wisdom will encourage us to face our personal challenges with renewed hope and confidence.

Dr Tony Bates
Clinical Psychologist, author of *Breaking the Heart Open*

OCTOBER 1973, ST BRIGID'S HOSPITAL, BALLINASLOE

For 11 days, I had lain there in a straitjacket, strapped into a hospital bed surrounded by steel rails. I was heavily drugged and having to battle hard to preserve some fragile sense of myself. It was dark; I hadn't a clue what time of the day it was, but the lights were on, which told me it was late evening, maybe night-time.

I felt alone, forgotten by the world outside the walls of that hospital. I was drifting in and out of sleep. A nurse appeared at my bedside, leaned over the rails and whispered kindly, 'Breda, how are you? Are you okay?' She bent down, coming closer so she could hear me. All I could say was, 'Please, phone this number. Tell my parents what is happening to me. Tell them what they're doing to me.'

Kindness was rare in that world; she stood out. Everyone else had curtailed me. Forcibly injected me against my will.

They had put straps across my tummy, then iron rails on the sides of the bed, as if I was going to go anywhere in a straitjacket.

Being in a straitjacket is beyond imprisonment. At least in an ordinary prison, you have the freedom to walk around. The freedom to eat your meals. I was totally restricted. I couldn't even move my hands. Even going to the bathroom was at their discretion – they decided the time, brought the commode, lifted me out of bed, put me back in again.

The nurse replied with a troubled look, saying, 'I can't do

that. I'll lose my job if I do that.' I pleaded with her using my eyes.

I was desperate. I could hardly talk; I was heavily drugged. I knew I couldn't say another word, but I stared at her, silently begging. After that, all I could do was hope.

Part One:

THE TWO ARROWS

INTRODUCTION

In the 23 years I spent in and out of psychiatric care and five psychiatric institutions in Ireland, from 1972 to 1995, nobody in that profession ever asked me, 'What happened to you?' I've always sensed that this was the critical question that would have made sense of my struggles and helped me form a more coherent sense of identity.

Instead, when I turned to our mental health system for help, I was prescribed psychotropic drugs, given electroconvulsive therapy (ECT) and restrained in a straitjacket, which did more harm than good. To this day, I still experience painful side effects from the 29 ECTs, including tightness in my scalp and uncomfortable sensations throughout my body. Pulsating nerve sensations are constant companions.

I appreciate that medication, including tranquillisers and antidepressants, may work for some people. But for me, they didn't help. Once, a psychiatrist told me, 'There are four families of antidepressants. I've tried you on each one, but none has worked.' Who knows what prolonged doses of multiple drugs have done to me.

Until now, I've never been able to speak my mind. As a child, I was terrified to express the sadness, anger and confusion I felt over how I was treated, especially by my father. When, as an adolescent, I sought refuge in a convent, I lived in fear of the harsh authoritarian regimen I found myself within, which discouraged, to the point of outright forbidding, communication.

As an adult, I was silent in the face of a psychiatric system where speaking out risked my being viewed as 'difficult' and treated even more forcefully than I already was.

Medical treatments failed to cure my depression because deeper psychological issues remained unresolved. I was diagnosed, and drugged, but nothing below the surface was ever explored. Perhaps the most significant trauma I suffered growing up was believing I was unloved. Whatever attention I received was conditional on conforming to strict rules and expectations.

What does it take to recover from multiple experiences of shock and hurt and make the most of our lives – even when our struggles seem to be more than we can bear, and we feel painfully alone? Until now, I've never been able to make sense of what happened that left me tormented with anxiety, low self-esteem and repeated bouts of suicidal despair for decades. More importantly, I've never been able to say what helped me recover. This book shows why I felt the way I did and what it took to find the confidence and self-belief to face my difficulties and manage the hurt inside me.

Chapter 1

WHERE IT ALL BEGAN

Trauma changes people. When he finished school, my father, who grew up on a farm in County Tyrone in Northern Ireland, with three brothers and five sisters, joined the British Army. He fought on the front line in the Second World War. When given the order to shoot, people died at his hands. Like many others, his experiences of battle trauma left him feeling disconnected and distressed. When we were children, he never spoke about the war. At that time, counselling was not an option. It was only when I went into therapy years later and started watching Second World War films that I began to really understand what he had been through in the trenches living with such violence. How in the name of God could anybody be the same again after experiencing something like that? You couldn't. I realised there was nothing to forgive. He was a victim of circumstances.

My father was a heavy, stocky man, with a round face. He was a domineering male influence over our house. From as young an age as I can remember, my father was violent towards me. As a child as young as five or six, I would have been locked in the bedroom for extended periods. They wouldn't give me any dinner. As part of my punishment, I was denied food until breakfast the following morning.

After one of those beatings as a small child, I remember lying in the bed and trying to find one part of me that didn't hurt. At the time, I didn't see anything abnormal about that.

Most of the time, we were just brushing past one another, rather than having much of a relationship. I lived in absolute dread of him coming into the room, because I didn't know what was going to happen next, what was awaiting me. I was terrorised.

I remember one day sitting down as a child to read a book, which would have been a very rare thing for me to do. Out of nowhere, this figure appeared and swiped the book from me, saying, 'What are you doing? Stop wasting time. Get up there and do the housework.'

I can remember incidents where my father would leather me, and I would be able to see my mother standing over in the corner, not lifting a finger to help me. I was distraught, crying. Why wouldn't she do anything for me? Why wasn't she trying? I had to try and cope with it on my own. I think now it was male domination. Maybe she was afraid of him too? Either way it never felt like she was someone I could appeal to. The odd time, she herself would also become physically violent towards me.

Times were also hard for my mother. She was born in a small village near County Tipperary's border, leaving home at a young age to work. She had six siblings, three boys and three girls, and also grew up on a farm. Money was scarce. People depended on slivers of land for a livelihood, and the children helped with the work from a young age.

My mother had never received affection from her own mother. We sometimes visited the family home in Limerick when I was a teenager. It was old Ireland – the fire, the turf, baking the bread. My grandmother was always cloaked in all black, a silent figure. I never saw one word pass between her and my mother.

In turn, my mother never hugged me, or showed her love physically in any way, but she didn't see any harm in that. I never remember seeing love between my parents either, our home was a constant battleground for rows between them.

I was born on 20 April 1949, in Holles Street Hospital, Dublin, the eldest of my family of seven siblings.

Growing up in a house of such chaos, there was no relationship between us children. It was a case of everyone trying to get through each day. There was very little lightness or play in our childhoods. When I was a youngster, the word 'survival' would not have been in my vocabulary, but now I can see that that's what I was just desperately trying to do. Survive each day. We did the best we could.

I was three months old when my parents emigrated to England. I travelled to London in a wooden orange box. My early years were spent at 36 Bavaria Road in North London. A severe attack of pneumonia meant that I wasn't expected to see my first birthday.

One of my earliest memories is of being left in my cot when I was very little. My parents were obviously making love. I could hear all these sounds. They frightened the living daylights out of me; I thought he was killing her. How could I have known what was happening. I had just been plonked in a kind of cage.

The Second World War had blighted everyone's ideas of a decent life. Poverty was rampant. Butter, tea, sugar, jam, cheese, eggs, milk and meat were scarce, and every family had a ration book. Our home was a three-storey dilapidated building. The place felt damp and cold. I found out much later that my father had bought the house to renovate the building and lease it to tenants. I can still see my father stepping down into the basement of our house after a long day at work. His face black and sooty, his clothes ragged and torn, the look on his face frightened me.

Gradually we filled the house with 16 lodgers. Mammy had to cook for all of us. One evening, I sneaked into the kitchen at the end of the corridor and stood against the back wall. She was bent over a low, deep, white sink with her sleeves rolled up. This was the first time I had seen so many dirty pots and pans. The surroundings were dark and gloomy. I wondered how she managed to cook there. A few weeks later, I remember her becoming very ill. She was coughing up blood and was diagnosed with a lung disease.

Looking back now, I can see that, like many women at the time, my mother was struggling with the burden of domestic life, and the dominant male presence in our house. My father was a heavy drinker, and probably spending a lot of their money on alcohol. I remember walking to the shop with her one evening, her grabbing me roughly and showing me a loaf of bread, saying that was all we had to live on for the week.

I think the circumstances of her life were very hard. In her way, she was trapped. Seven children. The expectations from my father on her, and on us children, as to the work he expected us to do, were colossal. He was working around the clock, and he expected all of us to do the same. Life was very hard for many women then. Now, I understand more about what her life was like, but as a child you cannot comprehend this. And she expected me to carry out a Trojan amount of housework, as if I, as the eldest daughter, was an extension of her.

Today, I see the happy, smiling faces of parents with their

children on their first day at school. Everyone wants to make this day as memorable an occasion for the children as possible and a fun-filled day despite the tears.

In the 1950s, post-war, life was very different. On my first day at school, I grasped my mother's hand as we entered the building. The place was packed. All I could see were towering adults above me. I held onto my mother for dear life, but when I needed her most, she let go of my hand and vanished. I looked back to see if I could see any sign of her, but she was gone. I was alone in a world full of strangers.

I remained motionless in the corridor, terrified. Everything was a blur. After some time, I felt a grown-up's hands on my shoulders from behind. I was guided into the classroom and brought to a desk in the front row. That afternoon, we were told to fold our arms on the desk, put our heads down and sleep. That made no sense to me. How could anyone sleep on a hard wooden desk?

Later, I glanced around the classroom. The other children had their heads down and were busy with their schoolwork. I continued to stare into space, not knowing what to do. I felt desperately out of place. The teacher came up, smiled, bent down, and, after a few kind words, showed me pictures from a nature book. I couldn't believe my luck when she said, 'Would you like to take the book home with you?'

There were moments when my father showed an entirely different side of himself to me.

I remember him bringing us one Sunday afternoon in London for a trek through the forests around Hyde Park. I was in my element as we meandered around the trees and windy paths. On another sunny afternoon, my mother brought a chair to the courtyard and gathered us around her to read a story. As I gazed at her, I thought she was the most beautiful person in the world. The fable she read fired my imagination and transported me to a different world.

My father was a member of Knights of St Columba, a lay organisation of Catholic men dedicated to charity, unity and fraternity. He was immensely proud of this. Once a year, there was a big ball, and my parents dressed up for the occasion. My father wore a dress suit and a dicky bow for the event, while my mother wore a glamorous dress. I was in awe at her long white gloves stretching beyond her elbows.

My father was a great dancer, and I love dancing and music. One evening when I was about 11 or 12, a waltz came on the radio. He took me in his arms, and we glided gracefully across the floor. I wished that precious moment would never end; I was in heaven. He loved tap dancing, and I dreamed I'd be able to dance like that one day. Fred Astaire, Frank Sinatra, Ginger Rogers and Gene Kelly were among his favourite artists. He also loved Bridie Gallagher, an Irish singer from Creeslough, Donegal.

One Christmas Eve, he lifted me high, put me on the top bunk of the bed alongside my brother, and taught us to sing the Christmas carol 'Silent Night'. I felt loved in a way that I never had before. I waited in vain for a repeat the following year.

In those moments, he was a totally changed man, but I do wonder in retrospect about the influence of alcohol on him at times. Was he merry and bright because he had been drinking, rather than it coming from a natural, loving space? He was a constant drinker. As alcoholism advances, maybe the violence advances too? He was in pain himself.

Sometime later, my father became a delivery man for builders/providers. During the school holidays, he used to stop by the house to pick me up in the van. I loved that time alone with him and would look forward to it. He was a different man. One day, as we drove along, he told me what life was like in his school. The headmaster entered the room every morning with a cane underneath his arm. With head held high, he strode to the teacher's desk. He dipped his hand in a box and took out a straight pin. If he couldn't hear the pin drop on the floor, each child received four or five strokes of the cane on each hand.

When I was nine, my mother enrolled me for piano lessons. Music would later become my lifesaver. Neither of my parents played any kind of instrument. I don't know where this idea came from. There was an old piano in the house when we moved in; somebody might have said it to her.

My teacher, Miss Gertrude M. Hales, lived nearby in North London. She was a kind, middle-aged lady. I was shy, sat quietly at the piano, and did what I was told. Now and then, she played along with me on the higher piano registers. That's when I played my best and enjoyed the lessons most.

One day, as I was about to leave, she reached up to the shelf, took down a jar and handed me two sweets. I will never forget the thrill of that moment. Thanks to my mother's safekeeping, I still have her end-of-term reports. They consistently describe me as a 'diligent little girl whose progress has been most pleasing and satisfactory'.

Chapter 2

GROWING UP IN THE SHADOW OF TRAUMA

Every family has its ups and downs, and we were no different. The Second World War had left my father with deep emotional scars. As a child I lived in fear of his dark moods and bizarre violent outbursts. To escape unhelpful emotions and painful memories, he often drank to excess.

One lunchtime, I was sitting at our wooden table with lodgers on either side. I could feel my legs dangling below me. All of a sudden, my father entered the room. I had just finished eating my first boiled egg in a cup, or so I thought.

I noticed he couldn't walk straight. He shouted, 'Finish that egg!' I didn't know what he was talking about. He came nearer and yelled, 'I said finish that egg!' What was I to do? Surely he didn't expect me to eat the eggshell! Like a giant hovering over me, he gave me a clout across the ear, grabbed the spoon, picked up the eggcup, and began scooping out something white. I hadn't realised that there's far more to an egg than the yolk, that there is a white as well.

He was livid and struck me so hard that I jumped off the chair and ran out of the room. He chased after me up the stairs into one of the bedrooms and leathered me. I backed into the wall as I kept begging him to stop, but he was on a rampage. I crouched in the corner, trying to protect myself, but to no avail. I ended up on the floor in convulsions, crying. He stormed out of the room. I was left numb and in shock.

Late that evening, I crept back into the dining room with nowhere else to go. An elderly gentleman was sitting in an armchair before a small fire. I tiptoed around the table, and with a kind smile, he opened his arms and invited me to sit on his lap. Normally a child would be apprehensive of a stranger, but I could tell he felt sorry for me. It was a bit like the nurse all those years later when I was in a straitjacket, I could just sense he cared. Here was someone reaching out to me.

I scrambled up and snuggled into the warmth of his clothes. I don't know how long I sat there but I felt safe and loved. He just happened to be there. I was fortunate. It was the first time I felt cared for.

In school, I struggled socially. As a seven-year-old, no one wanted to play with me in the yard. I couldn't understand why. Now I think, if the circumstances at home were so dire, which they were, there were probably no facilities to even have a bath. Did I smell? Also, I would have had no social skills. My siblings and I had never had the chance to develop in that way. I see my grandchildren now, playing and chatting with one another. I had none of that experience, so I wouldn't have known how to relate to other kids. I was a timid little mouse. And yet craving to belong.

One day, like a thunderbolt, a flood of strange, frightening body sensations overpowered me as I stood in the yard. My head felt tight like a balloon about to burst. It was a panic attack, not that I recognised it at the time – all I knew was that something scary I had never experienced before was happening to my body. I didn't know what to do. I stood there motionless, terrified. All I could think was, *I can't keep standing here alone.*

I have to do something. That's when I came up with my ingenious plan.

That evening, I took money from my mother's purse to buy sweets for the schoolchildren. *If I hand them around in the playground, they'll like me,* I thought. I kept that up for two or three days. Even though my heart pounded every time I dipped my hand into the purse, I had to do it. There was no other solution. The next day, in the yard, the children circled, pushing one another to get at the sweets. I was the centre of attention.

I was careful to try to ensure that I wasn't caught, but one evening, my mother caught me red-handed. All hell broke loose. She chased me around the table until she grabbed a hold of me. Her hands came flying towards me in all directions. I covered my face to protect myself. I pleaded with her to stop hitting me and kept telling her I was sorry. I tried to explain why I had taken the money, but she wouldn't let me get a word in edgeways.

Terrified of what my father would do if he found out, I begged her not to tell him. She did.

That evening, he charged into the bedroom. Roaring and shouting, he banged the door shut. I was too young to know any different, and when he called me names too painful to recall, I took every word to heart. He was my father. I looked up to him. When he started hitting me, I shrivelled up into a ball. I had no means of escape and wished I could disappear. Yet, he kept beating me even with tears streaming down my face.

By the time he left the room, my skin was bleeding and stinging like hell. There wasn't an inch of my body that didn't hurt. My mother was nowhere to be seen. I had nowhere to turn.

I could never make out why I deserved the punishments. For stealing the money, yes, but surely one punishment was enough. I had no voice. I felt that I didn't count. Nobody cared. When I returned to the schoolyard, I looked on in dismay as the other children sprinted all over the place, having great fun. Why did nobody want to play with me?

Growing up, the Catholic Church was an authoritarian, overbearing institution in our lives. My initial real experience of so-called God was my First Confession when I was seven. The teacher looking after it scared the living daylights out of me as she explained the rigid rules. She said that telling a lie in Confession was the very worst sin you could ever commit in your life. The way I survived was by sticking to the rules, in school as well as at home, so I took this very seriously.

First Confession and First Communion were the same weekend. It was a big dark gloomy church, all the children in a line. A nervous wreck, I was wracking my brains; how many times had I been disobedient to my parents. I had decided this would be my confession, and came up with this magical number: 99.

It came to my turn, and I went into a dark box. I told the priest, this is my First Confession, these are my sins. Then I blurted out that I was disobedient to my parents. When I came out of that confession box, I was in a kind of trance, struggling to deal with the stress of lying to the priest. All the rest of that day, I was eaten up with remorse and guilt, but there was no one I could talk to.

My mother helped me put on the white dress the next day. I felt unworthy of it, that was probably one of my first experiences of playing a part, like an actress in a film. I had no other way of coping. But I was acting.

It came to the First Holy Communion Mass. I just knew it was so wrong of me, evil of me, to be doing this, but what choice had I? I went through the motions. Sitting in my seat afterwards, I thought, *I am the only child in this church that Jesus didn't come to, because my soul is black.* I smiled in the photos taken later that day, but the smile was false. The guilt was eating into me.

A few months later, I still felt guilty about the money I had stolen from my mother's purse, so on my way home from school one day I went to Confession. Terrified of the dark confessional, I knelt and struggled to say the prayer we had been taught. 'Bless me, Father, for I have sinned …' I froze. An awkward silence followed.

Somehow, I got the words out: 'I stole money from my mother's purse.' Silence. Then, in a cold, stern voice, the priest replied, 'You cannot be forgiven until you pay the money back.' I left the confession box in tears. I had no way of replacing the coins. We didn't get pocket money. I was too young to get a job. There was nothing I could do. A dark, oppressive cloud hung over me, and the fear of the priest's pronouncement stayed with me for a long time.

My father and mother were rigidly attached to the rules of the Church. We would all be marched down once a month on a Saturday evening to Confession, an act I always found very stressful. It was a mortal sin in that time not to go to Mass on a Sunday. We'd all have to dress up in our best clothes, the ideal family to all outside appearances. At that time the priest would say the mass with his back to you, and it was all in Latin. For small children, it was extremely boring, but you just had to stay quiet and still in your seat.

My father would sing along with the hymns, and something about him would change. He enjoyed it. I loved that part of it.

Sometimes my parents and siblings would attend Mass on Sunday mornings but leave me behind to clean up the house. One morning when I was 12, I was dashing around to make the beds and tidy the rooms upstairs before returning to clean the kitchen. Halfway up the stairs, the front door opened. I froze. They were back.

Downstairs was still a mess. My father's temper exploded. He chased me into the front room and beat me with his leather belt. I collapsed on the floor with my hands and arms curled around me and pleaded with him to stop. He didn't. In the middle of his tantrum, he shouted, 'Spare the rod and spoil the child,' and struck me even harder. My mother stood like a statue nearby and did not attempt to intervene. I could never understand how she could watch and do nothing. At the time, it was very upsetting, but I have wondered since if she too was scared of my father.

Days later, Mammy told me we were moving back to Ireland. The day we left London, I stood outside the front of the house wondering how we'd all fit in the same car. Just at that moment, another car pulled up. We tumbled in. When we arrived at Holyhead, we headed straight for the pier and boarded the Stena Line ferry.

I was excited and couldn't wait to explore the ship, but my mother had other plans. She dropped the baby in my arms and told me to mind him. I kept my head down and remained in a bad mood for hours, which I couldn't shift. The following morning, I cheered up. When I got myself up on deck, dawn was breaking. I was intrigued by vivid colours and ever-changing patterns.

Daddy went to drive the car off the ferry while we disembarked by foot. Soon, we were on our way to Limerick. My parents had bought a small grocery shop with a family home attached, but there were some legal issues, and we couldn't move in yet. With nowhere else to live, we stayed with my aunt and uncle and their eight children.

They ran a busy farm. A large herd of cows had to be milked, and pigs, hens and chickens had to be fed. I couldn't have been happier when my aunt asked me to help her collect the eggs. My daddy's sister-in-law, Mary, always had time for me, and I loved being around her. In the kitchen, I watched her at the long wooden table, fascinated by the agility of her fingers as she made soda bread and kneaded the dough. She always had a lovely smiling face. The atmosphere in their house was so different to mine, and my cousins were always good to me, warm and friendly.

The first couple of weeks in my uncle's home were lovely, but gradually I began to feel very stressed. One morning, halfway down the stairs for breakfast, I was stopped by overwhelmingly awful sensations in my body. A tension that hadn't been there before had crept in. I found living under the same roof with so many people – four adults and all those children – difficult. I longed to tell someone the effect it was having on me. But I kept my concerns to myself. Talking about how I felt to one of the adults around me never felt like an option.

I see now that I was experiencing panic attacks. On several occasions, I woke in my cousin's bed, paralysed by intense feelings and sensations. For a couple of minutes I thought I was losing my mind, my grasp on reality, but I was terrified to let anyone know. I needed help, but I was afraid to say anything. The last thing I needed was for my cousins to think I was weird. I struggled out of bed and carried on with the rest of the day. Once the anxiety had been tripped in me, I couldn't enjoy my aunt and uncle's family home anymore, so I was delighted when we heard that the papers had been signed, and we could move into our new home, with the shop, my parents' new business.

I was excited, but that was short-lived. The minute we moved there, it was nightmare upon nightmare upon nightmare. Desperately trying to get the business to work, my parents were barely managing to make ends meet. Ferocious arguments between them were common. They fought about money and my father's heavy drinking; he was drinking to excess all the time. Thirteen by now, the eldest of seven children, I would watch them from the top of the stairs through the bannisters, scared.

Life at home was misery. In addition to attending school, I was expected to do housework, mind my siblings and work in the shop. The *Judy* and *Bunty* magazines I sneaked up to my bedroom were my go-to and any Enid Blyton books I could access. The Famous Five novels featured the adventures of a group of young children. I loved getting lost in the stories. On an odd Saturday, I escaped into the city shops to look around. It was great to get away.

I hated having to get up at half five or six to open the shop at 6.30, but I had no choice. When my mother or father told me to do something, I jumped. We all knew better than to disobey. The business's survival depended on the early morning trade and being there to catch shift workers on their way to Shannon Airport. I was the only one behind the counter, and when a queue formed, I always became nervous. I blamed myself if customers had to wait.

Every morning, I would enjoy a sense of freedom upon leaving the house, but once I got to school, I would feel this panicked sense of urgency about wanting, but not knowing, how to make friends. Not relating to anybody was a constant strain. I was a lone soul just doing what I was expected to do and what was expected of me, but so unhappy. I remember walking around the streets of Limerick and just longing to be part of a group.

After school, I would dread having to face back into home. My mother invariably called me into the shop to serve customers. I brought my schoolbag with me and tried to finish my homework. Some nights, I couldn't leave the shop until I had all the money in the till counted and the float was set up again for the morning.

At school, my strong English accent meant I was different from everyone else. I could also see that the girls in my class already had their circle of friends. Once again, I found it hard to fit in, feeling almost shunned. I did make one friend, and she invited me to her house a couple of times, but I didn't know how to relate to people. I used to find it an awful strain. I would be on edge not knowing how to talk to her. I was lonely, but had never learned how to socialise, nor know how to relate to people my age, and would end up a nervous wreck.

Irish was a compulsory subject for the state exams. I had never learned the language before, and the school arranged grinds. I liked the teacher and looked forward to the lessons. That was a break in the clouds.

When the school term ended, we went north to visit my daddy's family. After a long drive we were welcomed with open arms. I loved being there. My daddy was always happy on these occasions, although it was always drink, drink, drink. I used to dread the drive up, because of the number of pubs we would visit on the way.

One night, I woke up with a start. The music was loud and clear. I jumped up, ran to the top of the stairs, and peered below. People were gathered around the hearth playing accordions, fiddles and tin whistles. Various people sang their party piece while everyone else joined in at the chorus. There was an outburst of clapping and cheering. I sat there, taking it all in.

When our holidays were over, we returned to Limerick. One afternoon, I happened to be with my father in the sitting room when, for the first time, he began to talk about battles he had fought in. He picked up his army jacket, which I had never seen before, and showed me the medals he had received for service in the British Army. He moved over to the dresser, picked up a framed photo of himself and a comrade in army uniform, and looked steadily at it. I could tell that the photo meant a lot to him. I had never had this kind of conversation with my father before.

Now that I was a teenager, my father no longer beat me. There were times when he was still violent towards my youngest brothers – if they stepped out of line, he would give out angrily, often hollering, roaring and shouting at them like a madman.

At times he would smack them with his open hand like someone out of control – but no longer me.

When summer ended, I resumed school and my duties in the shop. Saturday mornings, I tackled the storeroom, even though I resented not being free to live my own life. Saturday afternoons, I had to bring the 'travelling shop' around the City Home, a hospital for older people down the road. Some of the wards had a stench that turned my stomach. I saw rows of older adults sitting on chairs in dark wards with nothing to do.

We were living a ten-minute walk from the city centre. Occasionally, when life became unbearable, I played truant from school. I felt ostracised at school, the tension at home was difficult, the hard work helping to run the shop exhausting. I remember seeing *The Ten Commandments* in the Savoy Cinema and another time, *Ben Hur*. I loved getting lost in the stories but having to face back into the harsh reality of life got to me each time.

Perhaps the most frightening thing to happen to me was being sexually assaulted as a young teenager by my father's best friend. I don't think my father had many friends, just drinking buddies, but he took a shine to this man. He had this amazing smiling face. When you saw him, you'd kind of light up yourself because, on the outside, he was so happy. He put forward a fun-loving image. To begin with, I enjoyed seeing him coming into the house because he was breaking through the atmosphere and the tension.

In our house, there was a hallway between the kitchen and the living room, then a door out into the shop. One day when I was 14, around two or three in the afternoon, he came in as usual. Everyone else was out of the house or in the shop working. I left the kitchen to go through the hall and he followed me.

He pinned me against the wall. I didn't know what was going on. I was so naïve. He proceeded to grope my body and my breasts. When he tried to kiss me, I managed to turn my head away. I had no means of escape; his body was too strong against mine. I felt so vulnerable, this hefty bulky man, and I couldn't move left or right, just yank my head trying to dodge him. It was awful.

That happened three or four times. Another time I remember running and running around the rectangular table trying to get away from him, and he caught me. I had no voice. I was paralysed. There was no one I could tell. I was frightened out of my life that if I mentioned it to my mother, she would rubbish it. If it got to my father's ears, there would be another explosion, outrage. How dare I say that. I would not have been believed. And I would have been punished for saying it. All I could do was try to ensure I was never alone with him in the house.

I grabbed every opportunity to cycle to my uncle's farm to escape my home environment. There was always a warm welcome waiting for me. I was in my element when my aunt brought me to feed day-old chicks, hens and pigs.

When my uncle needed help to save the hay, our entire family joined him in the meadow. Daddy was happy out in the open air, throwing forks of hay up on the haycocks. As youngsters, we had great fun trampling them down. We all gathered around for something to eat when the work was done. My aunt had brought a large basket filled with sandwiches and flasks of tea. Those were lovely days.

Daddy was more often than not angry and agitated about something. But he was a different man in the open countryside. His face relaxed. Nature brought him home to himself. He loved growing shrubs, flowers and trees and showed me how to propagate them. He liked having me around when he gardened. Guiding me around the flowerbeds, he pointed out the different flowers. Once, he picked a Lily of the Valley and passed it to me. His expression spoke volumes. He was in awe of the flower's delicate beauty. To this day, I owe my love for gardening to him.

I longed for my mother's love but could only relate to her superficially. She had her own worries. She always appeared to be unhappy, stressed and anxious. As a young teenager, I had no idea how to help make her happy. Both of us probably felt lonely, but neither knew.

My mother's health was deteriorating. The only decent break she had from the shop was her weekly visit to the hairdresser. After some time running the shop, my parents were audited by the Revenue. Strangers descended on our home for three consecutive days and poured over ledger books, accounts and receipts. I had never seen my father so broken. Everything my parents had worked so hard to build was snatched from them. These were such dark days. They were left virtually bankrupt, and the business eventually had to be sold many years later.

We were shocked but not completely surprised to hear that Mammy had to have major surgery to remove her lung. A couple of days after the operation, I found my daddy sitting at the table in the kitchen with his head in his hands. When I asked, 'Will Mammy be all right?' he looked at me with tears and awkwardly assured me she would be okay. That day, for the first time I saw how much he loved her.

When she recovered, I confided in her that I had a vocation. I wanted to be a nun. I sensed that was the last thing she wanted to hear, but I knew she wouldn't stop me. I was 15. As I had already attended the Salesian Order secondary school in Limerick, it was just a matter of formality to be accepted into the convent. The order had a noviciate in Brosna, Birr, County Offaly.

I had *conveniently* got a vocation. For me, the idea had formed as a means of escape, from the strain of my life in Limerick, the loneliness in school, the fraught atmosphere in my home, the abusive attentions of my father's friend. It was during an ordinary school weekend retreat that I had come up with this bright idea. During those days away I had thought, *This is my way out, this is my escape. I can get away from all that.*

I didn't realise for ages after I entered that there are stages to becoming a nun. Being an aspirant for two years is a bit like an apprenticeship. Then you are accepted into the order as a postulant for a year. Then you are a novice when you take your temporary vows of poverty, chastity and obedience. For the next six to nine years you are called, for example, Sister Agnes. Your new name is given to you by the order. Perpetual profession is for life. You become a permanent member of the institution – in the case of the Salesians, a lifetime member of The Daughters of Mary, Help of Christians.

At the time, my experience of the church was as an austere place. I went to Mass because I had to. We were marched down to Confession every single week. I hated it with a passion, found it terrifying. But it was a way out from the stresses of my home life.

My parents were not happy about my plan, but when the long list of items I needed to bring with me came through the post, my mother supported me in every way she could. I wanted to speak to my siblings about my plans, but they didn't share my excitement. I was the big sister; I was abandoning them, but my suitcase was packed and I was ready to go. The responsibilities I had been shouldering would now be dumped upon some of my younger siblings. I didn't realise this at the time. I had a hunch, but I wouldn't let it near me.

Chapter 3

IN SEARCH OF AN IDENTITY

Convent life in Brosna, County Offaly, run by the Salesian Sisters, was far from what I expected. Now aged 15, I had hoped for a nice life. I did not get it. Talk about from the frying pan into the fire. A shrill bell rang out each day at 6.30 a.m. We jumped out of bed, dressed quickly and lined up like soldiers at attention. The school was housed in a huge, intimidating building, surrounded by fields.

We marched to the refectory, bound by the rule of silence, and ate breakfast. Daily chores were conducted in fear of the nuns. They were very stiff and stern, regimental, a distant authority. Everything was clockwork. You would never be asked how you felt about something or were you okay. You might as well have been in the army; it was so regimental. Like at home, there was a total lack of kindness, and an expectation of heavy domestic work. I remember being on my hands and knees, polishing the tiled floor of an enormous hallway, terrified of missing even one black scuff mark.

On Saturday mornings, we helped with household chores. There was also gardening to be done. The afternoon was spent pulling out large patches of weeds. The flowerbeds had to look pristine before visitors arrived.

I recall the afternoon we were sent to the fields in our long black dresses to dig out mangels for the cows with our bare hands. My fingers stung and felt like icicles. I was angry that we were treated like that, but what could I do? One didn't dare protest.

Now and then, on a Saturday afternoon, a nun escorted us on a long walk, and even though special friendships were forbidden, we were allowed to have a few words with our companion. Apart from short recreational periods, we girls were forbidden to speak to one another. To break this rule was regarded as a sin. You were supposed just to be in communication with God – whoever God was; I never had a clue.

Life in the convent was all about power and domination.

Attending school during the week was a welcome relief. I liked being in fifth year. One morning, I was writing in my copy when, unexpectedly, I was called out of the classroom. The Intermediate Examination results from my previous school had arrived in the post. The nun scanned my results and acknowledged that I had passed every subject. But then she added, 'You are weak at Irish. You will have to stay back and repeat the year. Follow me.' Numbed, I walked down the corridor obediently without knowing what to expect. She led me to a different classroom, full of faces I didn't recognise. Suddenly, I became an Intermediate Certificate student again. That tore me asunder inside. It was so cruel. I had worked really hard, I even got Irish despite having grown up in England. And then just to have this towering figure standing over you, and you feeling totally diminished, as they are telling you what they want you to do. I had been happy and content in my class. The feeling of having no power within your own life; it was a bizarre world we were living in.

The first Sunday of every month, 2 to 4 p.m., was visiting day. Mirrors were forbidden, but we found a way around that. We stood behind a glass door in our black dresses and checked our reflections to see if we looked okay, even with our embarrassing haircuts (a short, straight line across the back and a short fringe across the forehead). Had we been found out, we'd have been in big trouble. Why? Because we had been perceived to be guilty of pride. I vaguely recall nuns standing on a pulpit in the refectory, admitting to a sin they had supposedly committed that day. I had severe reservations about the practice.

The monthly visits provided two hours of bliss when we could wander the grounds without supervision. During the Leaving Certificate year, my mother told me that my father hadn't spoken to her for two years after I entered the convent. He blamed her because I had decided to leave home and become a nun. This person that he could depend on to be there, doing all this work, and keeping everything ticking over was gone. Now the responsibility to make it work was fired back on them, because I had played a major role in keeping everything at least manageable. I was a domestic slave, cooking meals, cleaning, helping to run the shop, keeping the house going while my mother did her time in the shop.

When our visitors left, we had to hand over biscuits, cakes, sweets, and any gifts received. We never saw them again.

At times I pretended to be sick to escape the unbearable lifestyle and spend a few days in bed. I wasn't really physically that unwell; looking back, these were times when the mental strain got too much. I had little to do during the day except read schoolbooks and drift off to sleep. My meals were brought to me at a specific time each day; apart from that, I saw no one. I found the isolation painful. Sometimes, I struggled to stay in touch with reality, especially when I woke after sleeping long hours during the day and at night, as I had nothing else to do. I was a young teenager, in bed all day, isolated in a dormitory, curtains around my bed, nothing to pass the time, no visitors. No one ever asked if I was okay, just meals delivered at the appropriate times, and that was it. An odd time a nun took my temperature, but ultimately I decided when I was well enough to get up. When I literally couldn't stand it anymore, I just had to pretend I felt well again and push through as I always had. This was the beginning of a decades long cycle where I would become overcome with distress, seek retreat, but then feel forced to pretend I felt better in order to escape a situation where the right care was not being provided.

On those occasions, I sometimes felt I was losing my mind. I forced my eyes to focus on objects around me: the white curtain surrounding the bed, the rails holding them, the walls, and the dormitory itself as far as I could see. Slowly, I came back to myself.

Re-entering the daily routine was difficult. My legs would feel like jelly as I went down the stairs again, afraid I would not reach the next step. The sensations in my body were frightening. I couldn't think straight, it was as if I had been drugged (I hadn't). It was pure determination that I would get to the bottom of the stairs. I remember wishing I had somebody to talk to.

These episodes were a kind of breakdown. I wasn't functioning the way I was supposed to. It was dangerous, staying in bed for five, six, seven days, for hours on end, not sleeping properly at night because I had been sleeping through the day.

The only time the others came to the dormitory was to go to bed. The girls in that part of the convent were aged 15 to 18.

After 18 you went on to be a postulant. Everything was done in silence; we weren't allowed to talk to one another, there was no talk during the day, *ever*, except when you were in the classroom, and you had to answer questions. But there was no such thing as saying, 'Hello, how are you?' to the person beside you. It was total silence. We would not even catch eyes with each other.

On one occasion I had to go to the dentist in nearby Birr town. That was a big thing, because it was an escape. I was brought in a car. I got a partial denture on top, because some of my teeth were missing. Just to get to live in a day that was different was thrilling. The devastation then at having to face back into it was heavily felt.

What I now recognise as panic attacks happened frequently. Without warning, tremors of fear would take over my body, and my head would feel as if it was about to explode. The thought popped into my mind: *If anyone in the room sees this, they'll think, 'She's crazy.'* I closed my eyes, kept my head down, and hoped no one noticed.

I stayed at that convent for three years. I thought if I could stick it out, I would gain a sense of identity in becoming a nun. That didn't pan out.

I ask myself now: Why did I put up with situations like that? Why didn't I leave? The answer is, I couldn't bear going home. I believed that being a nun would give me a feeling of purpose.

There was also my passion for music. In Brosna, I was again able to avail myself of weekly piano lessons. By the time I reached my Leaving Certificate year, I had done grade eight in the Royal Irish Academy of Music exams and could play in school concerts.

I also played the piano accordion, bass drum, and various string instruments in the school orchestra.

But I was brutally unhappy there.

I was 17 when my 'spiritual formation' began in earnest. I became a postulant. That entailed getting up at 5.30 a.m. to meditate and pray before mass. We were given a copy of *The Imitation of Christ*, a handbook on the spiritual life by Thomas à Kempis. As a young teenager, I found the wording strange and scary. During a monthly meeting with my Superior, I asked, 'Who is God?' In an angry voice, she replied, 'God is a mystery. Don't ever ask that question again.' God was to be feared, never questioned.

By February of my Leaving Certificate year, I could no longer take convent life. I knew I had to get out, I couldn't stand it another second. I was 18, and cringed at the thought of taking poverty, chastity and obedience vows. I went to the Mother Superior, knocked on her door, shaking all over. I found the courage from somewhere to say, 'Please, I want to leave.' She replied, 'No. You have a vocation. You cannot go.' Three weeks later, I tried again. With a cross look, she said, 'Anyone who puts their hand to the plough and looks back isn't fit for the kingdom of God.' That was like punching me in the stomach. When I went back the following month and begged, this time even more tearful, she admonished me, saying, 'If you go against the will of God, your father who has angina could die from a heart attack. You will also be putting your family's business at risk.' I left the room in floods of tears.

Forbidden to confide in anyone apart from the Superior, still I took a chance. My piano lesson was due, and I told the teacher.

Talking to her like this was strictly forbidden but I was desperate. I had to risk it. She listened silently as I spoke through tears. That day she said little, but when I was still visibly upset the following week, she asked, 'Do you believe that God can speak directly through the priest in Confession?' I nodded. 'Go to Confession, then, and tell him you want to leave and see what he says.'

As nervous as I could be kneeling in the pew the next day, I somehow forced my legs up and went into the confessional, knelt, and told the priest I wanted to leave. He asked, 'Why do you want to go?' I said, 'I don't know; perhaps it's just that someday I'd like to get married.' I held my breath. The silence was striking. Then, I heard him say, 'I give you full permission to go. Tell your Superior.'

You could have given me an Olympic gold medal I moved so fast. I felt so empowered, probably one of the first times I had ever felt like that. I had got control of my life back. I ran up the broad stairs to her office like I was floating on air. I knocked on the door and heard her say, 'Come in.' This time, I sat in front of her desk with a strong sense of one-upmanship, announcing, 'The priest told me I can go.' To my pleasant surprise, in a mellow tone of voice, she encouraged me, for my own sake, to stay until the end of the Leaving Certificate examinations. Although waiting for even one more hour in the place when my body was in such an indescribable state felt like torture, that made sense. I decided to put all my attention on my studies.

History was my weakest subject. I was expected to fail the exam. As we lined up outside the examination hall, I noticed two officers standing outside the door. One held a stack of honours papers, the other the pass version. From out of nowhere, I thought, 'I'm going to fail, so why not fail on an honours paper.' When it was my turn, I walked up to the officer on the left-hand side and took the honours paper.

Finding myself sitting at the desk in the examination hall, I glanced through the paper. I couldn't believe my luck. There was a question on Feudalism. It was the only topic I had learned by heart. I knew bits and pieces of the others and wrote whatever came into my head. After the exam, I took it for granted I had failed. No one was more surprised than me when the results came out, and I got honours.

When the exams ended, my mother arrived to take me home. She had a disappointed look about her. Perhaps she had been looking forward to having a nun in the family. Three years of being cut off from the outside world had taken its toll. There was a strained silence in the car. I was nervous about going home, not knowing how I was going to be received.

When we got home to Limerick, I hoped my family would be glad to see me. Not so. My worst fears were met; I might as well have been invisible. That really hurt. Everyone went about their business as if I wasn't there, ignoring me entirely. My father never came near me. I didn't belong.

Before leaving the convent, I overheard that my music teacher had left the order before the state examinations. I found that hard to believe. Not once had she said that she was going. Now it made sense why she gave me her family's phone number when I told her I was leaving the convent after the Leaving Certificate exams. I understood from her it was in case I ever needed someone to turn to. She had been a place of refuge. One day, feeling painfully alone, I decided to reach out; I picked up the receiver and phoned. Her mother, a very kind person, answered. I learned that my teacher was now living in Dublin.

Her mother arranged for us to meet the following day in O'Connell Street. I jumped on a train to be there in time. She was smiling from ear to ear when we met. I found it strange to see her in civilian clothes, but we went to a café and talked as if we were the only two people in the world. It felt entirely natural. She was concerned about the hardships I had endured in the convent.

That night I stayed in a B&B quite near O'Connell Street. I can vaguely recall eating breakfast there the following morning and having a shower to look my best. Time dragged as I tried to fill in the hours before I headed back to meet her again. I read a book, the title of which I can't recall. I was on edge, jittery; I had butterflies in my tummy.

That afternoon, I strolled back to O'Connell Street. I couldn't wait to see her again. I noticed her coming, but something was different. Her attitude towards me had changed. I took this as a sign that she didn't want me around. I made up an excuse to get away. 'I'm sorry, I can't stay. Something has come up at home, and I need to get back.' Despite the awfulness of the situation, I kept hoping she'd ask to see me again. She didn't.

With a terse goodbye, she turned and was gone. I had never felt as insignificant or alone in my life. I kept peering after her until she vanished from sight. My body was rigid, but I couldn't stay there forever. I'm still not sure why her behaviour changed towards me. I turned and began the long trek back to Heuston Station. I cried the whole way, feeling more isolated than ever.

The only place I could go was home, but I remained on edge and felt out of place. A couple of days after the Dublin trip, unable to stand the tension, I went for a walk. I couldn't believe it when I bumped into Gay. A few years older, she had been a novice in the same convent but left the order a few years before me. We were both surprised to see one another and reminisced about bygone days. Her experiences of convent life were similar to mine. She understood what I was going through. That was all it took to steady my nerves.

Gay told me about a summer job teaching English to international students in the secondary school Kylemore Abbey, County Galway, telling me, 'Apply, you'll get the job.' When I phoned, I was hired on the spot. I left home the following day. I settled into the Abbey and enjoyed my work. The Benedictine sisters couldn't have been more pleasant or friendly towards me.

I also applied to Cork University to study for a Bachelor of Music degree. I didn't speak to my parents about my plans, they came entirely from me. One day in Brosna, walking down a corridor during my Leaving Certificate year, I had asked myself what it was I would want to do if I had the choice. I knew instantly: music. Music was the only thing in life I was interested in. It had been my salvation. A plan began to form in my mind.

I hadn't known I needed a Leaving Certificate in Latin to be accepted onto the course. I was shocked when I opened the reply and saw my application had been rejected. I broke down crying.

My new boss, the headmistress of the school, a Benedictine nun, rounded the school corridor at that moment, and spotted me in distress. She was kind and, much to my surprise, came up with the ideal solution. 'We'd be delighted if you could stay here for a year and teach music. You can study Latin with me and sit the Leaving Certificate paper next June. We'll pay you for teaching music. Board and lodging are free.' Who could ask for more?

I found I loved working as a music teacher, both in following the school curriculum in the classroom and teaching private piano lessons. However, there wasn't a time when I wasn't on edge as I found it so excruciatingly difficult to relate to people. I did my best to explain things to the students, while at the same time being painfully aware of my inability to have a decent conversation with anyone. I tried hard to come across as normal but the strain I was under ate into every fibre of my being. I never understood why. It's only in recent years I see my social skills were practically non-existent.

Towards the end of the school year, I saw one of my piano students to help her to prepare for her grade eight exam. Midway through the lesson, she became upset and told me about her terrible time at home. She was worried because our piano lesson was her last chance to practise. 'There's no way I can play the piano at home. It's not even safe for me to be there.' I replied, 'There's a spare bed in the dormitory where I sleep; perhaps you could stay there the night? I'll check with one of the sisters. That way, you can practise as much as you want, and I'll give you extra time.' We met 20 years later, and she couldn't thank me enough. She insisted, 'You saved me from despair.' I had no idea.

Shortly after, I was invited to work as a receptionist in the Kylemore Abbey Visitor Centre for the summer. I needed money to pay university fees, so it was an ideal opportunity to save, but I would have enjoyed the work more if I hadn't been tortured by the dark thoughts that kept going around and around in my head: *I'm not good enough. I don't deserve to be here. Tourists would benefit more if a person better able to do the job were in my place.*

On 21 August 1969, the Leaving Certificate results were delivered to the Abbey. There was an incredible buzz as students gathered to share the day's excitement. I held my breath as I opened the envelope. To my delight, I had passed the Latin exam. Now, at last, I could go to university.

Chapter 4

LOOKING FOR ANSWERS

Short in savings for the first year of music at University College Cork (UCC), I got a job as an au pair, which involved light housework and keeping the house clean. I took a bus to the outskirts where the family, two adults and three school-going children, lived. They welcomed me into their home. The next three weeks were about settling in.

One afternoon, in the front hall, I was cleaning, lost in my world, when suddenly I realised that the university term was about to begin and was opening soon, and I didn't know where to go. I dragged myself out the front door to find out.

I was now aged 20. I had been in a bad state for days, on autopilot. My distraction around when my classes started was a symptom of this. I was living life in a complete daze. I knew I had to get the au pair work done regardless of how I felt as I had nowhere else to live and no money to go anywhere else.

I went about my duties in a mechanical way, drifting from one job to the other like a zombie barely in touch with reality. My frantic thoughts circulated around my head: *I have to keep up. I have to get the housework done, clean the bedrooms, make these beds and hoover the house or I'll get fired.* I lived in fear of being found out as not what I appeared to be on the surface. I didn't know what was wrong with me, just that I was finding it extremely difficult to live each day.

When members of the family showed up, I forced myself to speak in a normal, natural way. But that was far from how desperate and pathetic I was feeling. I tried to answer any questions I was asked around the dinner table, but mostly I just sat there, unable to communicate with anyone.

I felt terrible. My body was struggling with an inability to put one foot in front of the other. I was at such a low ebb, but I didn't think I was physically ill. Physical illness to me was when you go to the doctor when you have something definite – a flu, measles, something wrong with your heart, or you've broken a bone. I knew that these sensations were something totally different, but I didn't know the cause, and I didn't think it was treatable. I didn't know what mental health was at the time. I didn't have the words.

On my first day of university, I took the bus to Cork city. I jumped off and walked the rest of the way to the university.

I stood mesmerised when I arrived at the sizeable square quadrangle in front of the university and saw a massive building surrounding me. The infamous Honan Chapel caught my attention, and I wandered over to look closer. The church, built in 1916, was famous for its Romanesque architecture and nine Harry Clarke (1889–1931) stained-glass windows. From inside the chapel, the windows were magnificent. I had to tear myself away.

Outside, I was struck by the volume of students dashing back and forth. I stood and looked on in bewilderment. Nearly overwhelmed, I considered turning around and forgetting all about studying music at the university, but that didn't seem feasible. Going back to Limerick wasn't an option. I forced myself to keep going.

The Music Department was located in an ordinary house. The room on the ground floor where we attended lectures accommodated a small number of students. I was glad of that and always sat in the front row to block myself from interacting with others. I was still nervous around people and didn't know what to say. My concentration was poor during lectures, and I had to force myself to listen and take notes. The moment the lecture finished, I left the building without speaking to anyone.

We were a class of nine. Two girls went out of their way to be friends and occasionally called at the house to invite me out. I went a couple of times but generally avoided their company. I was remorseful for not reciprocating their friendship, but I was shy and didn't like social contact. I didn't realise that three years of living like a hermit in the convent had impacted my ability to form relationships.

Professor Aloys Fleischmann (1910–1992), the head of the faculty, had an aura around him that commanded respect. Twice during my three years at UCC, I went to his office looking for answers only he could provide. On both occasions, I worked myself into such a state that I became tongue-tied and struggled to get the words out. I had been telling myself, *Who am I to be alone with such a prestigious figure?* But he was courteous, kind, and helpful.

I'm also honoured and privileged to have studied under Seán Ó Riada (1931–1971), the founder of Ceoltóirí Chualann, a traditional Irish music group. Sadly, on 3 October 1971, he died a few weeks before our graduation. Shock waves rippled through the university at his untimely death. When I play the organ in church, I take every opportunity to play his world-renowned piece, 'Ag Críost an Síol'.

In my first year, I attended various lectures on composition, harmony, musicology and traditional Irish music. A European language was obligatory. I chose Italian as I had some knowledge from school. Throughout the semester, I had to force myself to keep going. I had no energy. Every step felt like an effort. In my mind's eye, I can still see myself, head down, pressing forward along the Grand Parade in Cork, desperately trying to get to the Music Department on time.

In general, the family I was staying with were friendly, and we got on well. That was until alarm bells went off in my head when I noticed the mother was drinking alcohol to excess. I also saw her husband coming home from the pub a few times drunk. Having grown up in the home I did, I found this especially difficult to witness, and concern for their children weighed upon me. Seeing small children in that situation was heartbreaking.

The odd weekend I went home. I once mentioned that I liked dressmaking in school. The next day, my mother returned from Limerick city with a second-hand Singer sewing machine for me to bring to Cork. It was an unusual but very welcome show of care from that quarter.

I was good at dressmaking, and I remember walking down the Grand Parade one beautiful sunny day proudly wearing a dress I had just made. My mother had been sending pocket money. Otherwise, I wouldn't have been able to afford the material. The hobby helped me to relax and enjoy life. After that, I was back to my studies.

The Bachelor of Music degree requires a high-performance standard in an instrument of choice. Mine was the piano. In the host family's home, there was a piano in the sitting room. Every morning, after I had finished the housework, I sat down to practise. My classmates seemed to be far ahead of me in their playing. I worried that I might never reach the required standard.

Frédéric Chopin, born in a small village near Warsaw, Poland, was my favourite composer. His music resonated deeply with me and transported me to a place beyond my typical everyday experience. I felt drawn to the military style behind some of his compositions, for example, Polonaise in A Major. I could sense the power in my hands as I played the deeply resonating chords.

While attending university, I had a piano teacher who was a renowned concert pianist and teacher of classical music. I couldn't believe my luck when she agreed to teach me. She was polite but distant. I made great strides under her guidance, firmness, and close supervision. One weekend, I spent hours practising an intricate piece of classical music. I didn't give up until I had mastered every single note. I couldn't wait for my next piano lesson to play the piece for her. I expected great praise, but she scrunched her face in a frown and said in a cross voice, 'Is that all you think there is to music? Just the notes?' There wasn't another word spoken. I left the room in tears, shattered. I wonder now if I was unable to play with the feeling she demanded, given how shut off I was from my own true feelings. At the time everything I did was mechanical, whether it was practising the piano, learning a new piece, or my work in the house I was living in. All of them were duties that had to be performed.

Today, when I play the organ in church, I relate to the lyrics of the hymns, and in a heartfelt way I express how much the words mean to me through the notes I play. I'm always surprised and delighted when parishioners come up, thank me for the lovely music and say how much my playing means to them. One night, the priest said that my music helped everyone pray. I was astonished. While it took me years to figure out where my piano teacher was coming from that day, now I appreciate the importance of playing from the heart.

In early June 1969, the host family invited me to go on holiday with them for a week to County Mayo. While there, I tried hard to fit in and be my best. Behind the mask, I was sad. I was lonely. I did enjoy the beauty of nature. I can still see myself sitting cross-legged on a steep embankment, looking out on a world where time stood still. Those feelings had always been there, I was so used to it by then I just thought it was normal. I didn't realise things could be different.

I asked the family to drop me off in Galway the day we left. From there, I travelled to a small coastal town in Connemara, searching for a summer job. I doubted anyone would take me on, but I needed money to continue my studies.

I was a nervous wreck as I made my way into a prominent hotel. The proprietor, an elderly lady, had a commanding presence. I couldn't believe my luck when she offered me a job as a receptionist. My role involved welcoming guests and checking them in to the hotel. I was welcome to avail of free accommodation in the staff quarters.

Every morning behind the reception desk, I remained unsure of myself. The thought of having to relate to people scared me. I was happier doing administration work and taught myself to type to write up the menus.

One late evening, near the end of the season, a man entered the hotel who I vaguely knew. He walked up to the reception desk and started to chat me up. I was astonished when he asked me out on a date. I didn't want to go and tried to put him off by saying, 'I'm not finished work until 9.00 p.m.' He replied, 'That's okay; I'll return then.' I was taken aback but agreed to meet him at the main door. Saying no didn't feel like an option.

I finished work, dashed upstairs to change, came down again and saw him waiting in the foyer. I wasn't sure what to do or say next, but he escorted me to his car. We sat in and exchanged pleasantries. He looked straight ahead and switched on the ignition. Before I knew what was happening, he revved up the engine and sped off down the road.

To my utter disbelief, he swerved into the church car park. Seconds later, there was a loud, grinding thud. I froze. He began to curse and swear. Numb with shock, I didn't know what to do. The car was at an angle. His side was higher up than mine. Angrily, with the engine still switched on, he twisted the wheel back and forth until the car landed on the tarmac. He glanced at me with a disturbed look and said, 'I'm sorry.'

My first date. I was in shock. I didn't know what to expect. I thought I had to respond when he reached over to kiss me. He became overpowering and managed to coerce me into the back seat of his car roughly. I was naïve. I didn't know the facts of life. My mother hadn't explained them to me, beyond one day in the house in Limerick, when I was upstairs in a bedroom, she had looked at me and brusquely said, 'One of these days you're going to start bleeding from the top of your legs.' And then she was gone, leaving me completely confused.

Before I realised what was happening, he forcefully pulled down my clothes. My instincts told me to run. Panic-stricken, I pushed up hard against him, got myself out from under his body, reached out over the seat, grabbed the passenger door handle and ran for my life.

I exploded into tears and could hardly see where I was going. When I reached Main Street, the night unnerved me even more. Petrified, I glanced back to ensure he wasn't coming and kept running. There wasn't another person on the street, not even a bicycle on the road.

After a restless night, I woke to an onslaught of painful sensations in my body. I struggled to get out of bed and stood on the floor in a blank, vacant state, shell-shocked. Something told me I needed to inform someone, but everyone around me was a stranger. I could only hope I'd make it through the day. Decades later, I found the courage to return to the church car park to see where the car had landed. The tombstone was on the right-hand side, up near the church. I froze, then walked away.

Chapter 5

FALLING APART

On 6 October 1969, I returned to Cork to begin my second year at university and resume my work as an au pair. At the house, conditions had deteriorated. Every single room was in disarray. Things were strewn everywhere, and the place was filthy. I worked hard and got it back into shape. After that, I did my best to steer clear of family involvements, but there was no escaping the children's mother either falling around in the hall or trying to get up the stairs drunk before collapsing into bed.

Two neighbours told me on more than one occasion that I could move in with them. I was relieved to hear they knew how bad things were. But how could I leave three small children to fend for themselves? I couldn't. One morning, I came down for breakfast, and there wasn't even a bowl of cereal for them to eat. Upset, I grabbed my purse, ran out the front door, and rushed to the shop to get groceries before they went to school.

After a while, I got fed up waiting for buses and walking the rest of the way to college, so I bought a second-hand moped with money I had saved up. I was excited as I kickstarted the engine for the first time and headed into town. I found it breathtaking as the cars whizzed by, the wind on my face, but I stayed in my lane, and all was well, the whole world going by me. It was a rare occasion when I was in touch with myself, living in the moment. The sense of freedom was exhilarating. It reminded me of when I was a teenager in Limerick, when things would get too much at home and I would cycle out to my uncle's farm.

During my second year, an older student, a renowned uilleann pipe player, checked now and then to make sure I was okay. I pretended I was. He invited me and the rest of our class to his house for a music session one evening. When I arrived, other guests were going through the front door, and I slipped in unnoticed.

I gazed in awe at the buffet on offer – all sorts of delicious foods spread across a large wooden table. We helped ourselves, stood around, and ate away to our hearts' content. Again, I kept my distance from the others. We sat in a group when everything was cleared out, and the music began. A beautiful atmosphere filled the air as the playing of the uilleann pipes wafted through the room, and all the other musicians discreetly joined in, transporting me to another world. There was a second, similar evening. There was a magic to them that carried me forward.

When I had arrived in the city, I ran into a Benedictine nun doing a Bachelor of Arts degree in Cork. She had taught me the Irish harp when I was teaching in Kylemore Abbey. She offered to continue with lessons. I also learned how to play the pipe organ in the cathedral that semester.

One day near the end of the university term, I was sitting in front of the massive organ, practising the pieces, when a frenzy of uncomfortable body sensations hit me like a bolt out of the blue. It was as if my body was seizing up. I couldn't play. I was shutting down. I felt the tension building in my body, which was trembling, I swung around on the organ seat, hoping to find some connection with the tabernacle below. I felt nothing. I turned back to the organ, distraught, grabbed my music and left.

At the time, I was under intense pressure to get to know the pieces well because I was sitting exams soon. On top of that, the stress of living with alcoholics meant it was all just becoming too much. That day, I thought I had lost my mind.

Out in the street, people brushed past me. I was in a bad state and couldn't stop crying. I remember two women giving me a quick side glance as if to say, 'What's wrong with her?' I buried my head in my chest and kept going. I didn't realise at the time that this was a panic attack. I certainly had no understanding of where this emotional distress was coming from, or what had originally caused it. I had never heard of things like mental health, or mental illness. But I had learned as a small child to push through, ignore how I was feeling and just keep going. As far as I was concerned that day on the street, I had *no option* but to keep going. It wouldn't have even occurred to me that these were emotions, connected to what had happened to me in my past, which were building up inside me, needing to be dealt with.

I went back to my room and hid, hoping no one had seen me. It was such a secret life. Nobody knew how I was feeling, I was always putting up a mask. I was terrified to do anything else. I couldn't afford to let the family I was living with see that I was in a bad way. I often thought to myself that I'd make a brilliant actress, I became so good at it. There was no alternative. Opening up would have meant falling apart, which would, in my mind, have meant annihilation. What do you do? Collapse on the street, with everyone around you?

I was desperately trying to hold on to some bit of sanity for myself. Against the odds, there was something in me that was striving to keep intact. Anything else did not feel safe.

One thing that kept me going was looking forward to Sunday nights and being in my bedroom for the Radio Luxembourg Top Twenty. There, I could let the world go by as I waited excitedly to hear which singles had made the top three.

At some stage, I joined the university choir. I enjoyed the rehearsals but felt weird the night we performed at the Cork International Choral Festival. In my mind's eye, I can still see myself, second row back in the middle, appearing to be the same as everyone else but torn apart inside. At least 50 or 60, if not more, choir members were on stage, but I felt like an outsider. I stood like a statue, motionless, uninvolved, struggling to open my mouth to sing. Professor Aloys Fleischman conducted the choir that night. The fact that I felt unable to confide in anyone about how I was feeling served to heighten my isolation.

Towards the end of May, the second-year results were out, and I had passed all the exams. I returned to summer work in the hotel in Connemara. I don't know what I was thinking, but on top of my reception duties, I offered to come in at 6.30 every morning to open the hotel and switch on the plugs for the heating, hot water, ovens, et cetera.

My intentions were good, but the strain of getting up early, day after day, took its toll. I was already quite fragile. I was afraid to tell the manager I couldn't do it anymore. I was scared of losing my job. I needed the money to continue my studies. When the morning shift ended at two o'clock, I went straight to bed, but the onslaught of unpleasant body sensations was unbearable when I got up again to be in time for work at four.

Day after day, the only solution I could find that enabled me to go back to work was to have a scalding hot shower. I didn't know what else to do. The season ended in late September, and in October of 1970, I returned to Cork for my final year.

My mother had been sending me pocket money every week, helping at a distance. I treasured this. It was so valuable, and I don't think I would have made it through college without it. And it was a small inkling that she cared about me, a rare feeling between us.

At the start of the new term, my parents offered to drive me from Limerick. On arrival at the house where I lived as an au pair, my dad parked the car across the road. I jumped out, rang the doorbell and held my breath. The children's mother opened the door. Instinctively, I looked over her shoulder, and what I saw made me shudder. I didn't need to look any further; even the hall was filthy. Clutter and dirty rubbish were lying all over the place.

I couldn't take it anymore. I turned and rushed back to my parents' car in tears. For two years, I had been dedicated to my job. I was shocked that no effort had been made to keep the place clean in my absence. I sat in the back seat of the car, engulfed in tears.

I managed to tell my parents about the two people who had said I could live with them. My parents offered to pay the rent, and I felt safe there.

Finally, I was free to focus on my studies, but my health didn't improve as I had hoped. I kept up appearances, but one

Sunday morning, disaster struck. I was going to the local church for Mass when I realised I had no energy. I couldn't go forward; I couldn't go back. I tried again and this time managed to keep going. By the time I had slipped into the pew a few seats from the back, I was just about managing to stay in control.

During Mass, the crippling boredom of remaining in one spot, regardless of how weak and in turmoil I felt, riled me even more. I knew the sensible thing was to get up and go, but I couldn't. I kept telling myself that the people behind me would be appalled if I left. I could imagine the whispers, the gossip. But in the end, I had no choice but to leave. On the way back to my digs, uncontrollable tears rolled down my face. I turned the key, slipped in the front door unnoticed, went to bed, and cried.

The following morning, I was up again to face the day. I always attended every lecture. In May 1971, as well as written papers, we had to perform three classical pieces on the piano in front of an audience. My head spun when I walked out on the stage for the piano recital; everything around me was a blur. I thought about leaving but imagined the shocked horror that would spread through the audience if I did. I made it over to the grand piano and sat on the stool. My hands shook, but I put my fingers on the keys, looked up at the music and began playing. Somehow, I got to the end. The audience applauded.

That summer, once the holidays began, I travelled to Connemara once more to resume work in the hotel. The proprietor called me one day and told me she had bought another hotel nearby and would like me to be the receptionist. I enjoyed reception work, but the owner asked me morning after morning to dust the lounges, which were full of small antique ornaments. Although I tried my best, I didn't have the patience for the work. I wanted to tell her but hadn't the courage to say how I felt.

On my days off, I visited my friend Bernie. We had first met when she came to me for piano lessons; she lived across the road from Kylemore Abbey, where I was teaching and living while studying Latin to get into university. Bernie is a year younger than me, and we had become friendly. On Sunday afternoons, we would stroll as far as Kylemore Bridge, sit on the wall and listen to a football match on her transistor radio. Her family welcomed me into their home and invited me to stay whenever I wanted to. They always treated me as if I was one of their own. She was the first real friend I had, and I felt comfortable in her company. Years later, as we celebrated her golden wedding anniversary – I played an electric keyboard during the renewal of the vows – I told her how good she and her family had been to me. 'Breda, what are talking about? You were like the sister I never had,' she replied.

During the summer holidays from university, I would sometimes go and stay with Bernie and her family at weekends. As well as the emotional struggles I was concealing from everyone, I was still shy and socially awkward, but Bernie used to encourage me to go to dances with her. I loved dancing, because my father had been a great dancer. All the time I was living with a mask, so ill inside, I was still trying to keep up with a normal life.

Around this time, I had my first boyfriend, but Bernie had to call me eventually to tell me that he was two-timing me. I was devastated. A few days later, Bernie rang me and said there's a dance tomorrow in Roundstone, would I come? I told her, 'No way, I'm finished with that.' She shot back at me, 'Please come. If you don't go, I'm not going.' I reluctantly agreed to go.

Walking out of the Abbey, dressed in a miniskirt I had made myself – the higher up the better – there was a car parked across the road. Bernie was going with Willie at that stage, now her husband. I noticed a guy sitting in the back seat. Annoyed, I thought to myself, *What? She's gone and flipping arranged a blind date for me.* I was ripping. And I wasn't a person who would usually get angry, but I was livid that night with Bernie, absolutely raging. But I couldn't turn back; I didn't want to cause a scene.

Begrudgingly, I sat in beside this man.

Bernie introduced me to Tommy. I was too mad at her to take him in. I didn't say a word until we got to Roundstone.

When we arrived at the hall, I dashed out of the car and tore in to get as far away from the others as possible. The band was playing. In those days, the men lined up on the left-hand side of the hall, the ladies on the right. I scooted over to the right as far away from them as I could go.

Some fellow asked me to dance, and I did. Then I saw Tommy coming over. He asked me to dance, and I couldn't be rude, so I agreed to go out on the floor with him, but I vowed not to say a word to him. And I didn't. He must have thought I was the coldest, most awful creature on this planet, because there was no response from me whatsoever.

The minute the dance was over, I returned to my place without saying a word to him. By the night's end, I was in better form and had started to hope Tommy would ask me up for the last dance. That was my better nature rising to the surface again. Luckily, he did, and I thought, *I'll be more civil this time, but there's no way I'm going out with him.* We danced, but things were still off.

Tommy by this stage had had enough of me. He had hoped to sit in the front and drive, but Willie had the keys and was already there, so he was forced to sit in the back again with me.

On the way home, I sat tight against the backseat window. Tommy sat as far away as he could on the other side. Willie began to drive mad fast around the corners, and Tommy and I were thrown on top of one another, which was exactly what our friend had intended. Each time, we jumped right back to our own opposing sides. In the end, Bernie turned around and said, 'Tommy, the worst thing she can do is slap you across the face.' I replied, 'Oh, I wouldn't do that.' Tommy told me later, 'Breda, that was the first sign I had that there was anything likeable about you.'

Eventually Bernie swung around and said, 'Will you two stop acting like children.' She leaned over the seat and pulled the two of us together.

We started going out as a foursome, travelling to marquees and hotels for dinner dances. The hotel provided a four-course meal followed by a night of dancing to a band.

I felt at home with these three people. I felt accepted, safe. To this day, Tommy and Willie, and Bernie and I are extremely close.

One Saturday night the four of us travelled 50 miles to see Big Tom and the Mainliners, a country and western band. Not for the first time, while we were out the negative sensations coursing through my body felt intense. I always hid what I was feeling from everyone because I thought no one would understand. I was jealous of other couples who had their health and were enjoying life. So much of my energy had to go into pretending I was well.

Three or four months down the line, Bernie and Willie broke up for a short time. I honestly thought that was me and Tommy finished as well. I felt bad about it, but I just thought that's life, as if I wasn't really deserving of something so nice. But that week, on the night Tommy was due to come over, I looked out the window of Bernie's house where I was staying, and I could not believe my eyes. There was Tommy's car at the driveway. It was the first time that I realised he really cared about me. Why else would he come over on his own? That was the opposite to everything I had experienced in life up to that moment. From that day on, I began to open up to him. I felt so at home with him, I could tell him things I had never mentioned openly to anyone.

On 9 November 1971, we drove to Cork for my Bachelor of Music graduation. The conferring was held in the Aula Maxima. I got caught up in the excitement when I heard my name being called out. I walked up to the podium to loud applause, where I was presented with my degree by the university's president. After the ceremony, we gathered outside in the courtyard for refreshments.

I moved away from the crowds and walked down a narrow path. The beautiful day and brilliant sunshine grabbed my attention. I had every reason in the world to be happy, but I was miserable. Everything around me felt unreal. I couldn't wait to get back to the car. I was overcome by an onslaught of unpleasant physical feelings I didn't understand. My body went rigid. I was afraid of losing control.

When I felt a small bit better, and the sensation was beginning to pass somewhat, I returned to my parents and Tommy. I longed to tell someone how I felt but was too scared that they would judge me.

After graduating from Cork, I moved to Galway to do my H. Dip and be near Tommy. I was living with a retired nurse, renting a bedroom, and I had access to the kitchen below.

One lovely sunny Sunday afternoon, Tommy asked if I would like to come and meet his parents. I had gathered along the way that that was a big deal. I said I'd love to. I wasn't well, but I had kept up appearances. Even though I had begun to confide somewhat in Tommy, he had no idea of the extent of my anguish.

When we got out to his house, I was welcomed with open arms. I sat amongst Tommy's large family, as they chatted and caught up. The atmosphere was magical to me. It was so relaxed, with laughter ringing through the house. I watched as someone came in and another person jumped up and gave them a hug. It was unlike anything I had experienced in my own home. I could see the love between them. I sat back and thought, *I want this for myself*. I didn't say it out loud, but every cell in my body was full of that idea. I had found something I wanted.

By this time, I knew I had to do something about my health. Since early childhood, I had lived through experiences of physical and sexual abuse, then three years of strict convent life had compounded my distress. Family relationships at home were strained. As an au pair, I had lived for two years in a house where both parents had alcoholism. I had been under constant stress while attending university. I worked hard in the hotel to impress everyone. I was almost raped, and no one knew. I badly wanted to talk to someone.

Even though I didn't have an appointment, I went to the university doctor in Galway. I managed to get in to her, and tried to explain why I had come, but she didn't have time to talk. I see now she was caught for time, but I wouldn't have realised that in the moment. I was desperate for someone to talk to. I said something urgently like, 'I don't feel well, I don't feel right.' She listened for a couple of seconds and then she started to write out a prescription. I had no idea why or what she was giving me. I thought maybe she was just writing down a good tonic. I took the bit of paper, thanked her and left.

I went directly to the chemist. That's when I discovered that as well as vitamin B_{12} injections to be administered by the hospital, the doctor had prescribed Valium tranquillisers. I panicked. Shocked to my core, I couldn't think straight. I broke down crying on the street. The upset was that I felt I was being written off as mentally ill. I felt that this was saying there was something fundamentally wrong with me that couldn't be fixed, but merely treated with medicine to keep things at bay.

It didn't feel right, but I did not know what to do. I wouldn't have realised at that point that everything I had experienced in life up until then was trauma. That word wasn't even in my vocabulary. All I knew was that I wasn't well. I wasn't in a position to associate what I had lived through with why I wasn't feeling well now.

I had struggled through in Cork for three years and had

managed to keep going, but now, doing my H. Dip, I knew my health was in trouble. I can still see myself walking along the road near the hospital after going to the pharmacy saying to myself, *I have to do something about my health.*

I was so upset that I dropped everything and hitched 50 miles to Clifden to tell Tommy. He was the only person I could turn to. Tommy worked in construction, and when I arrived, he was working on a house. I came upon him up a stepladder. He was totally taken aback too. 'Tranquillisers?' He couldn't figure it out either. Then he thought for a minute and said, 'The doctor must know what she's doing. Perhaps you should take them.' I felt uncomfortable but began the prescription.

Over the next few months this doctor treated me for depression with various medications, none of which helped.

Today, I appreciate that some people may need medication to settle them enough to explore their symptoms, but what's sad in my case is that it all stopped there. I was prescribed medicines without any word of explanation, or any further exploration into what was actually upsetting me. It felt as if I had been given a diagnosis, and things left there. Had the doctor had time to sit with me and allowed me to talk about the issues troubling me, I believe my life would have taken a different path. I suffered from depression, but it was the type of depression that was a natural outcome of what I had lived through. Because what person would not be depressed? What child could not be depressed?

I needed someone who cared. Someone who understood that my health had been impacted poorly because of what had happened to me. A doctor who, out of respect, asked me first if I would like a mild tranquilliser to help with symptoms as a temporary measure, and after hearing my story, perhaps realised that counselling, for example, would be of great benefit. What I wanted was someone to talk to, but that did not seem to be on offer.

Having treated me first with Valium, then antidepressants, eventually, the GP said she couldn't do anything for me and referred me to a psychiatrist working in St Brigid's Hospital, a psychiatric hospital in Ballinasloe, County Galway. She told me I could see him privately in his house near the hospital. It all sounded okay. I had no option, I knew I was unwell, what could I do? I had to follow through. I was 22.

Part Two:

UNHEARD

Chapter 6

THE PSYCHIATRIST

My first visit with a psychiatrist was a brief, ten-minute consultation. Most of it was spent taking down my basic details: name, place of birth, address, parents. It was all very matter of fact, surprisingly so.

Tommy came with me and sat beside me during the questions. At the time, it felt quite normal, like being transferred from one doctor to another, sent to a consultant, a specialist in what I might need. He prescribed Librium and said he'd see me again in a month. I was so disappointed at how short our appointment was, and that he never asked me what was happening at that time, how I was feeling or what had happened in my life that might have explained the symptoms I was experiencing.

We had travelled 60 miles to see this man. For what? Just another prescription for another antidepressant.

My gut was telling me no when it came to taking more medication, but I didn't listen to it. I didn't know about instincts at the time, I had too little sense of myself to trust my inner wisdom.

Tommy and I didn't really talk about it afterwards. I think from his point of view it was just taken as equivalent to a visit to the GP. Okay, they said to go here and so we'll do what they're telling us to do. That is how things were then. Questioning the doctors would have felt impossible.

Despite how I was feeling, I kept up with my studies and passed my exams. During the conferring ceremony in UCG, 21 July 1972, I was presented with my Higher Diploma in Education Certificate by the President of University College Galway, Dr Martin J. Newell. For me, the day was a matter of form. I could find no pleasure or excitement in the event. I was getting tired of pretending I was well when I was miserable behind the mask.

That September, I began working in Kylemore Abbey as a music teacher. I enjoyed the work, but my health was poor. I continued to see the psychiatrist monthly in Ballinasloe. Besides Tommy, nobody else knew I was going. I would have felt embarrassed to admit it, a sense of, *My God, is this what I've been reduced to?* But there was also a feeling of having no other way out.

Every month, Tommy would drive me down to visit the psychiatrist – I couldn't drive myself as I didn't have my licence yet. My health was a nightmare, a constant struggle. Looking back, I would have been in no condition to drive even if I had my licence, but I would have preferred to travel on my own. The shame I felt for being that unwell was something I wanted to hide. I found it very difficult to keep pretending I was just as well as everyone else.

Inwardly, I was distraught, barely ticking over, although somehow I managed to get through each day. Mostly, I felt in a severe numbed state, hoping against hope something would change and I'd feel better, but it never did. I wasn't tearful. I didn't cry, as far as I can remember. I didn't want to let on how bad I felt.

I religiously took what was prescribed. Something in me felt resistant, because I couldn't see any benefits from the treatment I was receiving, but you did as you were told. And I felt caught in a dilemma. I had to do something about my health. But the so-called help I was receiving wasn't making any difference whatsoever. I wouldn't have known anything about what is now called talk therapy. It certainly wasn't something I experienced with the psychiatrist. I assume the GP who had referred me had sent on the original diagnosis of depression, but he never discussed this with me, just wrote a prescription. When Librium had no effect, he switched to Surmontil and an antidepressant. When these medications didn't work, in December 1972, about five or six months into my attending him, the psychiatrist convinced me that the only choice was electroconvulsive therapy (ECT). 'Nothing is working. There's only one option left. Electric shock treatment.'

I knew nothing about it; I had never heard those words before, but it sounded awful. I can still remember my body recoiling when he said them. But you trust the doctors. I trusted that he knew what he was doing. He was the professional, the person who knew about these things, I believed in him from that angle. Not that I knew him as a person. But as a doctor. I trusted the profession. They know what they're doing, you go along with them – that would have been my automatic thinking. I knew how desperately unwell I was, that it had been going on for years, and that I needed to do something. What could I do? I didn't know any other options. They told me this was what would get me better again. So be it.

That psychiatrist put me through ten electric shock treatments. I have no recollection of them. For whatever reason, they are gone; I blotted them out. Recently, I had a strong flashback and can vividly recall being in a long ward like a dormitory during the weeks I was there. The beds were in a straight line stretching down further than I could see. There was a similar row across from me on the opposite side with barricaded windows rising above them.

My striking memory of that ward is how white, stark and clinical everything looked: white starched bed clothes, nurses in white uniforms, and white walls with no curtains around any of the beds.

What I do remember is that with those treatments I was gradually getting worse and worse and worse, to the point where I was unable to keep teaching in Kylemore. I had to give that up, which was devastating. It felt as if the ground was taken from underneath me. I felt like a nobody.

At the time, only Tommy knew about my mental health problems because he was there with me. I imagine Bernie and Willie got to know eventually because Tommy told them. I didn't tell my family in Limerick. I told no one. I was too ashamed and embarrassed. I didn't want people writing me off as 'suffering from my nerves', as people put it back then.

As things got progressively worse, the psychiatrist then referred me to St Patrick's Psychiatric Hospital, Dublin. I was very reluctant to go as an inpatient, but he persuaded me that 'the only way to be available to them' would be 'to stay a few days'. I felt uncomfortable and checked with him again that I could leave whenever I wanted to. He insisted that I could return home any time because I was going as a voluntary patient. I believed him.

*

On 5 December 1972, at 3.15 p.m., I was admitted to St Patrick's Hospital in Dublin. With money bequeathed by the author Jonathan Swift, it was founded a year after his death, in 1746, one of the first psychiatric hospitals in the world. Many extensions have been added since.

That day, the building struck me as horrific, prison-like. Dilapidated, austere, very intimidating. When we arrived, Tommy was ordered to leave almost immediately. That threw me, and I froze. I couldn't understand why they wanted him to go. I felt in a whirl of utter confusion. I stood motionless in the huge entrance hallway for a long time, like a statue, petrified, wondering what would happen next. Alone, at 22, my first time in a psychiatric hospital as an inpatient.

It would be February before they let me out.

I had hoped that I would hear about everything that would be done to help me regain my health and that I would be treated with kindness, compassion and respect. I'd also expected there would be a range of activities I could enjoy.

Instead, when a nurse arrived to take me to the ward, she said coldly, 'Come with me.' In the dormitory, she ordered me to take off my clothes and jewellery, put on my nightwear and get into bed. I wasn't sick enough to necessitate being confined to bed and felt humiliated and frustrated that I was being told what to do without any explanation. She made a list of my belongings and took everything away when she left. Almost instantly, I began to feel like a prisoner. It felt as if I was being punished, when I had come for help.

Many years later, in 2022, I obtained my medical records through the General Data Protection Regulation (GDPR), to help me understand what had happened while I was there and how the hospital staff had viewed me. Reading the notes all those years later was very tough. The language used about me felt degrading and shocking. But they were also a gift; they gave me a lot of information I either didn't know or had forgotten. In a way they gave me back my past. I felt they validated my story. What psychiatry did to me was there in black and white. Proof.

In going into a psychiatric hospital as an inpatient, I had wanted someone to listen to me and appreciate how specific experiences in my life had impacted my health. I believe that would have made a difference. Instead, my interactions with staff were entirely focused on psychotropic drugs and ECT.

> **File notes:** 5 December 1972. New patient admitted to room bed at 3.15 p.m. Pleasant and cooperative with admission formalities. Has been teaching in Galway for years, but recently has been unable to cope with classes or to concentrate. Charted for Laroxyl 25mg twice a day. Valium 5mg four times a day, and Mogadon 10mg at night. Good evening, tea taken. Settled and sleeping at the time of the report.

The following day, I was allowed up for breakfast in my pyjamas. When the meal was over, I walked the corridors and looked around the old-fashioned building, with its depressing walls, heavily locked doors, and nothing to do. I'd had enough. I wanted to go home, but I was trapped.

The psychiatrist in Ballinasloe had assured me several times before I left for the hospital that I was a voluntary patient and could leave if I wanted to. My gut had felt uneasy, and I had repeatedly checked with him that I could I leave when I wanted to. He was adamant, yes you can. I feel so angry about that. How could he not have known what was going on?

That first full day in St Patrick's, I went to the nurses' station and asked to leave. The nurse on duty responded with a cold and callous rebuke, 'No one in the hospital would discharge you.' That hit me hard.

I considered how I might get the authorities to change their minds. I soon realised you had to pretend to be well to get out. This would happen in every psychiatric institution I spent time in. I made a tremendous effort to appear well. I was pleasant and cheerful in my interactions with nurses. But my plan backfired. My attempts to appear normal were interpreted as a hypomanic state.

> **File notes:** 7 December 1972. On seeing the patient on subsequent occasions, the original diagnosis of depression (probably reactive in type) had to be amended to one of a manic-depressive state. Anxiety neurosis is also present.
>
> Predisposing factors to depression are an unstable environment during childhood, her university studies, wanting to force herself to do well as her parents were paying for her final year accommodation, her career as a music teacher, and the worry of the effect depression may have on her [upcoming] marriage. A nervous, anxious, conscientious personality subject to mood swings. The

day after entering hospital she developed a hypomanic state.

Suggestions for treatment: Having seen the development of the hypomanic state, the original treatment plan for depression treatment with Librium, Parnate or Laroxyl, had to be amended to possible ECT or Lithium treatment.'

It is with regret that I look back on my first week at St Patrick's Hospital. Had people recognised my agitation and allowed me to settle in my own time and speak about what had happened, I believe I would have felt cared for and safe. I imagine my mood would have naturally improved in a matter of days. Instead, I was confined to bed, and my distress was entirely attributed to a mental illness I could neither understand nor control. I felt utterly disempowered and demoralised. Despite my requests, they wouldn't give me my clothes back and I was kept in pyjamas.

I hate the phrase mental illness, because it is saying there is something radically wrong with you. And there's no acknowledgement in it of you as a person *at all*.

With each day, I became more withdrawn. My freedom to choose had been taken out of my hands. I had no option but to comply. I had very little social skills at that point in my life, so I had no way to relate to my fellow patients, but to pass the time, I did try to talk to them a little bit, but mostly I was very much a loner in St Pat's. I was terrified out of my mind. I kept to myself, kept my head down, desperately trying to get through each day as best I could.

> **File notes:** 8 December 1972. Bed Rest continued. She is sleeping for long periods. Remains anxious at times. Pleasant on approach. Helpful. Appetite good. Seen by Doctor … at 6.50 p.m. To discontinue Laroxyl 25mg twice a day for the present, till seen by Doctor … as she appears to be elated.

The nurse's reports confirm that I slept for long periods. Being confined to bed and medicated, there wasn't a lot else I could do. It all felt so unnatural. I became increasingly frightened of myself. When I was awake, I felt 'very restless' and had 'anxious periods', as my file notes recorded. But no one took the time to ask why. I began to feel more like an object than a human being. I kept hoping the next day would be better, but each day was just more of the same.

On 12 December 1972, the nurse's notes verified that I had received a letter from home containing some terrible news about a friend who had died by suicide. Naturally, I longed for someone to talk to, someone who would understand my grief. There was no such person to turn to. I asked, but not even the doctor was available that day. I coped as best I could.

As the weeks passed, the nurse's notes record: 'Mixing well with fellow patients.' I asked that my clothes be returned, but my request was refused. I was 22 years old and found it degrading that anyone could have that power over me. I often simply sat in the chair alone. The nurse noted: 'Not so talkative today. But remains anxious about herself.' My medication was increased to: 'Valium 10mg four times a day, Mogadon 10mg at night.'

Throughout my nine-week stay, a nurse would stand over

me until I swallowed the tablets. I appreciate that the nurse had to do her duty, and perhaps some patients needed that kind of supervision, but I found the practice humiliating. It was a severe blow to my self-esteem; I couldn't even be trusted to take a couple of pills.

On 13 December 1972, nine days after being admitted to the hospital, a nurse arrived with my clothes. Still confined to the ward, the nurse's notes describe me as being 'helpful'. I was allowed to attend a relaxation class. The next day, there was a lecture for patients on the stigma surrounding mental illness. I was excited after the meeting and planned that when discharged, I would do all I could to help people understand the experience of anxiety and depression.

I was completely drugged out from psychotropic drugs and my world was a haze. One afternoon, I was staggering along the corridor when a male psychiatrist approached. I had never seen him before. He came out of nowhere, stood in front of me, and said, 'You're never going to get better, unless you have electric shock treatments.' I froze and gazed at him in horror. It was like a cannon ball had hit me, the force with which he spoke to me, the fact it was an ultimatum, that I was in a public place. I was so ill from the drugs, which had made the situation I went in with a hundred times worse.

When he was gone, I grappled with his ultimatum and tried to find some way around it, but there was none. I was at a breaking point and realised that I would do anything to get my health back, even if that meant more ECT treatments. Reeling, I tried to make my way back to the ward, hand by hand gripping the walls. I was terrified. But what could I do?

I had already had ten unsuccessful ECTs in St Brigid's Hospital, Ballinasloe and they had made matters worse. Inwardly, I lost the grip of myself. I was less in control. It was like looking out on the world in a dazed state. I had no energy, doing the smallest thing, like moving from place to place during a typical day zapped the little energy I had. There wasn't a moment that I didn't feel wiped out.

But maybe this time round, ECT would work. I had no option but to trust that the psychiatrist knew what he was doing.

That day, I just about made it back to the ward. Later, the day nurse confirmed in her notes that I was 'restless, agitated and anxious over self and wanted something to do'. No notice was taken; I was left sitting there. There was nobody to talk to.

The next day, I was brought for ECT. Inside the door of the relatively small treatment room, I froze. My legs refused to move. When I was told to approach the bed, I had to cooperate. The medical staff were warm and friendly and helped me up. A mouth guard was put into my mouth, then a circular contraption was positioned over my head.

Two electrodes, contact points for the electric current to pass through the skin on the head, were placed on both my temples. Electroconvulsive therapy causes a seizure to bring about electric and chemical changes in the brain. I was given an anaesthetic and injected with Scoline, a muscle relaxant.

> **File notes:** 15 December, '72. Has just had ECT this morning. Feeling sleepy and is very confused. She felt well on the 12th till she got a letter from home containing some depressing news about a friend. Depressed again

on the 13th. She feels she hasn't had the opportunity to talk to a Doctor, which may hinder her progress.'

I was allowed out for a few hours when Tommy visited that weekend. The authorisation was given on condition that I'd be back 90 minutes later. I made the most of the time but dreaded returning to the hospital.

I asked Tommy to intervene so that I'd be discharged. When he didn't get anywhere with the nurse at reception, he requested to see a doctor. I stood a few steps back. As I listened to the conversation, I could tell Tommy was getting nowhere, and even worse, the doctor's arguments were swaying him. I didn't stand a chance.

I was now on Valium 10mg four times daily and Mogadon 10mg at night. Sodium amytal, a prescription drug used for its sedative and hypnotic effects to treat anxiety, epilepsy and insomnia, was added.

> **File notes:** 18 December. Attended relaxation classes, also P.T. classes today. Complaining of feeling anxious and worried about various things. Discussing other patients' problems with them. Tearful and complaining of feeling depressed. She was seen by Doctor. Sodium Amytal was ordered and given. More relaxed after same. Visited by cousin. For Scoline and ECT in the morning.

The ECTs continued. When I regained consciousness after my third, I couldn't move a limb. I found myself lying on top of the mattress, unable to do a thing. I recall thinking I was like a vegetable and wondering, *Is this me for the rest of my life?* With my eyes open, I had to lie on the mattress motionless for hours. I was helpless. Eventually, I drifted off to sleep.

When my eyes fluttered open, I noticed the Christmas decorations. Slowly, I turned my head right and then left. There wasn't a soul around. The hospital ward was deserted. *It's Christmas Day,* I thought. *That's why everyone's gone home.* I felt a profound sense of loss, a deep sadness. I literally couldn't move. I was trapped on the bed I was lying on. I had missed Christmas dinner with my family. I had no choice but to accept that was the way things were.

I am unclear what happened after that. A couple of days later, I was in bed when my aunt came to visit me. When she left, I asked to be allowed home for what I thought were the remaining days of Christmas. Permission was granted.

Emma, my cousin, who was travelling to Limerick, collected me. The nurse's notes describe me as 'excited to be going home'. At the nurse's station, Emma complied by signing on the dotted line. I caught snatches of her conversation with the nurse on duty. I thought Christmas Day was over, but to my utter astonishment, I gathered from what they said that there was still another day to go. I couldn't make that out, and everything inside me spiralled into agitation and confusion. How could I have got my dates so wrong?

At home, I felt drained and unwell. None of my immediate family ever came to visit me in hospital, over all the years, and that Christmas nobody asked how I was although they knew I was in Pat's. It was only when I read my medical records years later that I saw it was my father who had signed permission for ECT. That shocked me to my core.

I tried to put up a front for the sake of my brothers and sisters. However, family tensions, the demands of the shop business and my dad's heavy drinking tore me apart.

I returned to St Patrick's on 27 December in a 'very depressed and tearful' state, as the file notes record. I longed for someone to confide in, but there was no one I could approach. Later, I was informed that I was scheduled for more ECT treatment the following morning. By that stage, I think I was hardened to the outside world. You begin to repress the feelings, instead going stone-faced.

Fifty years later, I question the effectiveness of electroconvulsive therapy. In my experience, they were cruel treatments. At the time, my mood if anything worsened, and I was left for years afterwards with extremely painful constant nerve pain. After my fourth ECT in St Patrick's, the nurse's notes report: 'Good recovery from Scoline and ECT. Disprin tablets given for headache. Attended relaxation classes. Sleeping long periods. Pleasant and helpful.'

The following day: 'Up and dressed all day attending full routine. Complaining of feeling depressed and dull. Very anxious afternoon. For Scoline and ECT in the morning.' After my fifth ECT treatment: 'Tearful and complaining of feeling depressed. Seen by the Doctor. Sodium Amytal given at 2.00 p.m. For Scoline and ECT treatment.'

Sodium amytal is a central nervous system depressant that affects a naturally occurring chemical in the brain called gamma-aminobutyric acid (GABA) and controls excitability in the nervous system.* I still don't understand why I was prescribed such a potent drug.

After each of the nine ECT treatments, the nurse's notes record similar observations about depression: 'Complaining of feeling depressed and dull. Very anxious afternoon.' 'Tearful and complaining of feeling depressed.' I could never make out why ECT, which was supposed to remove depression, was not only proving ineffective but was adding to my suffering. The nurse noted that after my ninth treatment, I was still 'tearful and upset', and that even after sleeping for long periods, I 'remained depressed'.

I was also suffering blinding headaches, but initially I was afraid to speak up. I tolerated the ferocious pain until I could no longer bear it. Then, I called a nurse and told her I couldn't stand the pain in my head. She returned with two Disprin. I couldn't believe it. I was in severe pain. Why wasn't the doctor on duty called? Why wasn't the excessively high level of pain investigated?

There wasn't a moment during my stay that I didn't want to leave. I was there as a voluntary patient. I was 'free to leave' in theory, but I was weak and vulnerable without anyone on the medical team willing to listen and represent my wishes to the authorities. Being able to leave was never spoken about or mentioned when I was in those places. There was fierce opposition to asking. One wouldn't dare. The fear of being

---

* Raspolich, Joseph. 'Amytal Addiction.' Serenity at Summit, 24 Oct. 2019, https://serenityatsummit.com/barbiturates/amytal/. Accessed 1 Apr. 2025.

prescribed even stronger drugs because of being seen as 'difficult' ensured I kept my mouth shut except for those odd occasions when I found the courage in a gentle way to ask could I go home.

I should have been allowed each and every time I asked, but perhaps the nurses had been drilled as to how to respond and would have been brought to task had they tried to stick up for me. Perhaps their conditioning was so strong they had to go along with the authorities above them even though they knew it was all wrong. The fear of losing their jobs was more than likely another deterrent and strong reason to conform. I was afraid to speak out. I regret that now. But what I wanted didn't seem to count for anything.

> **File notes:** 5 January 1973. Bed rest continued. Depressed this morning but in better form this afternoon. Seen by the Doctor. Anxious to go on leave. Doctor ... refused same. She is very depressed because of the slow improvement in her condition. Attending relaxation classes. Allowed to have clothes and walk in the grounds.

It occurred to me that perhaps the deterioration in my health was related to the severe impact of drugs and ECT treatments on my body. I wanted to discuss this with my doctor as a matter of urgency. I asked a nurse to ask her if we could meet, saying 'I'm really worried what the medication and the ECT treatments are doing to my body. I'm not getting better, I'm getting worse.' She looked at me scornfully and said I was talking crazy nonsense. When the night nurse came on duty, I tried again.

She also told me frankly that I was being stupid. I felt intimidated and gave up.

At that time, I needed someone to take me seriously and try to understand what I was feeling. I needed someone to know that the distressing sensations in my body resulted from the many traumas I had suffered. Had psychiatry understood the root of my health issues, I would have been spared unnecessary pain and suffering. Nobody asked what had happened to me to cause such terrible anguish. I suffered two levels of pain. The pain of hidden, unresolved trauma in my body and mind and the pain of nobody 'getting' me.

During the sixth week of my admission, I was permitted to spend time with Tommy. I enjoyed the freedom of being with him. On my return, I pretended I was much better than I was in order to get discharged as soon as possible.

> **File notes:** 8 Jan '73. In good form. Up and dressed. Attended relaxation classes. To attend Group Therapy tomorrow. Helpful on ward. The patient both looks and feels good this morning and doesn't seem very much elated. She was out at the weekend with her boyfriend and felt well.

I'm surprised that the doctors and nurses viewed me as being in good form and didn't see through my pretence. That I 'felt well' is what I told the doctor. She changed my Largactil medication to Parstelin 10mg in the morning and 10mg midday.

There were really only three types of psychiatric medication. Tranquillisers, antidepressants and mood stabilisers. There are major and minor tranquillisers: Xanax, Valium and Lithium being minor, and Largactil was major. Developed in the 1950s, Largactil was a very powerful drug. It flattened people; they would use it also on horses. It was principally for psychosis. It was prescribed to people who seemed agitated, or psychotic or deluded. It had terrible side effects – people could appear with their jaw twisting, make funny movements – people who were taking it might look mad, and then could be further diagnosed with a mental illness because of the impact of the drug. It is not used anymore.

Parstelin was also a major drug. Also not used anymore, it caused severe liver and kidney problems. It was a heavy hitter antidepressant, not an anti-psychotic; it didn't have any tranquillising properties.

I know from my medical records that I attended two group therapy sessions that week. I can recall sitting in a circle in a spacious room and feeling overwhelmed as the facilitator went around the group and encouraged patients to share personal details of their lives. I have some recollection of a couple of patients who became visibly upset. I was troubled by what I heard but couldn't say a word. I felt it wasn't my place to speak out. I didn't feel safe enough to open up. After the meeting, I returned to the ward confused and frightened by the unpleasant sensations in my body. I couldn't think straight. I was distraught. Perhaps I wasn't ready for group therapy and would have done much better if I could have had a one-to-one session to clarify what I was feeling.

File notes: Patient is being moved to Ward 5 today. She is very active and alert, but this appears to be a sign of the patient's return to her normal personality, rather than a swing towards hypomania, as was thought earlier on in her admission. Still on Parstelin 10mg. Is participating in all hospital activities.

A few days later, the notes continued:

The patient had ECT (7th) on 17/1/73. She has been feeling depressed since moving to the new ward. She was still depressed on 18/1/73 and was to go out for the day with her boyfriend. She was home for the weekend, having had another ECT on 19/1/73 (8th). Still feeling depressed and required Sodium Amytal 3gm. stat. today.

On 23 January, I had my ninth treatment. The nurse's notes read:

Had Scoline and ECT. Satisfactory recovery from same. Became very tearful and upset after same. Complained of feeling depressed. Seen by doctor. Retired to bed at 3.45 p.m. Slept long periods till 7.00 p.m. Remains depressed.

I remained puzzled as to why, after all the medication I had taken and ECT treatments received, I was still depressed and finding it difficult to cope. The question in my mind was, *Why am I still feeling worse instead of much better?*

As a patient in St Patrick's Hospital, I remained at a loss to know why it was that whenever I saw my psychiatrist – who was polite, warm and friendly – she never seemed to listen. I sensed that something other than mental illness was at the root of my ill health. Deep down, I knew I couldn't be right when the ECTs and various medications I was on were making me feel worse by the day. I asked myself that question at one point: *Why are ECTs that are meant of get rid of depression making me feel even sicker?* I knew, too, there was something below the surface that wasn't being addressed. I didn't have words for that at the time. Now I know it was unresolved complex trauma.

In my ninth week of hospitalisation, I continued to pretend that my health was better than it was. I received permission to go out for the weekend with Tommy. In February, I was discharged on the condition that I would continue taking the prescribed medication – Surmontil, 25mg twice a day and at night, Parstelin 10mg in the morning and 10mg midday, Valium 5mg four times daily – and attend St Brigid's Hospital, Ballinasloe, for further ECT treatments. The choice was mine. I could agree to those terms and conditions or remain in the hospital. I agreed.

The day I left St Patrick's Hospital, I could barely walk down the corridor and held tight to Tommy's arm for support. I was scared I wouldn't make it to the main door. The consequences of showing any sign of weakness didn't bear thinking about. Regardless of how I felt, I had to appear normal.

The fact that my stay in St Patrick's had done nothing to improve matters is clear in notes from two years later, when I was admitted to St John of God Hospital, Stillorgan, Dublin. A medical report dated 25 May 1975 refers to my stay in St Patrick's Hospital over the last months of 1972 and early into 1973.

> Patient first went to Doctor ... in Ballinasloe with depression. She was treated with ECT and tablets. He sent her

to St Patrick's Hospital where she was again treated for endogenous depression with ECT and tablets and was no better when she came home – worse, in fact.

Over the years, I have felt angry at a psychiatric system that laid down the law to the detriment of patients, that treated me with brusqueness, ignored my appeals to talk to someone when I tried to express my fears over the side effects of psychotropic drugs and ECT treatments on my body, and failed to investigate the causes of my distress.

Had I been encouraged to speak about critical experiences in my life without judgement and fear of recrimination, I would have had a better chance of recovery. Sometimes, sharing unpleasant feelings and sensations with someone compassionate and understanding is all it takes to calm everything down. Emotions must be heard, acknowledged, and accepted before a renewed emotional balance can be reached.

During my nine-week stay in St Patrick's Hospital, I believed I had no choice but to suppress painful emotions as they arose. I didn't understand that I was making matters worse for myself and sabotaging my health.

As a child, I was too afraid to stand up to my parents and express my anger for fear of another beating or punishment, like being denied food, locked in a bedroom for hours, and not spoken to for days. As an aspirant and a postulant in the convent for three years, I didn't dare express anger over harsh treatment and forbidding rules for fear of offending a God I didn't know and being regarded as a sinner. I spent two years in Cork burying painful feelings as a young adult when deeply upset, as an au pair, over having to live with two parents who had alcoholism. The same pattern was repeating now.

Over time, I have allowed myself to express anger through writing. I would write repeating sentences that all began: 'I am angry because ...' and pour my grievances onto paper. Once, I ended with a note: 'I can't believe I've just spoken so openly and so honestly. Who is this person? I've never met her before. You're experiencing uncomfortable emotions that have a right to be heard.'

Recently, I wrote another note to myself:

> I hear you, Breda. You have a lot to be angry about. You've had to keep that anger tucked away for years as you were busy loving children, grandchildren, friends, fellow parishioners, and, of course, Tommy and his wider family. People needed you – and still need you – so much. Feeling angry about what happened long ago may have felt like a luxury you couldn't afford. But we deny anger at a cost to our health. Suppressed anger can be so disruptive in the body. It burns and bruises us.
>
> Accepting and allowing ourselves to feel what we feel is the most important thing we can do. As Dr Edith Eger wrote, 'You can't heal what you can't feel.'* Sometimes our strong emotions must be allowed to run their course before they naturally calm down. Recognising and befriending those parts of you that are angry is what your anger may need now.

* Eger, Edith Eva. *The Choice*. London, Rider, 2018, p.259.

You are hurt that no one 'saw' you for who you were at a time in your life when you badly needed to be listened to. What felt most vulnerable in you deserved to be heard and recognised for how painful it was. But you can welcome all of those feelings now and allow them to be part of your unfolding identity.

When someone did see and hear me, something healing nearly always happened. It made me feel that what I was experiencing was real. And that, in turn, allowed me to be the person I was, both fragile and robust, both victim and survivor. When another human being acknowledged that what I was going through was valid and understandable, my sense of self clicked back into place.

Chapter 7

WEDDING DAY BLUES

I'd always imagined my wedding and honeymoon would be happy times. That's not quite how things turned out.

I was someone who had grown up without love, or any close relationships. In Tommy, I had found a person who really cared for me. He looked after me, brought me out on dates, wanted my company. Even though I was sick, I had good times with Tommy, unlike anything I had ever known previously.

So then what happened was I became more and more terrified of losing him. Things reached a crunch point where I felt I could no longer take the risk of losing him. One night, out on a date, I said to him – I'm mortified about it now – 'Tommy, can we get married, will you marry me?' He was taken aback, but looked at me and said, 'Yes, we'll get married.' It should have been the other way around; it would have been nice if the traditional way had happened. I jumped the gun. If I had had my health, I would have waited. But I admire Tommy for doing it. He gifted me that certainty.

We were to get married on 30 July 1973. In the months leading up to my 'big day' I'd been taking my prescribed medications and attending Ballinasloe mental hospital for another course of electric shock therapy. St Patrick's Hospital had made the latter a condition of my discharge.

I would stay with my good friend Bernie after I attended these treatments. Whenever Tommy couldn't drive me the long distance because of important commitments, Bernie always did.

She remarked years later that I appeared to be drunk after each session, telling me, 'There was no coherence to what you were saying, you kept repeating the same thing over and over again to the point where you almost drove me daft. It was heartbreaking to see you like that. I was extremely concerned about what the psychiatrists were doing to you.'

Between St Patrick's Hospital and Ballinasloe, I was subjected to 29 ECT treatments in total, from September 1972 to May 1973. I had hoped they might help, but they never did, and I was left with terrible nerve pain and headaches. Instead my health continued to deteriorate.

No longer working in Kylemore, I had returned home to my parents' house in Limerick to focus on wedding plans, burying myself in what had to be done so I wouldn't have to think of anything else. Money was scarce, I made my wedding dress and the bridesmaids' dresses and offered to make my future mother-in-law's outfit. I designed and created the wedding invitations and made a three-tier wedding cake.

I drove myself hard. Wedding preparations were the only thing I had to keep me going in life. I took it for granted that I could push on, but early one morning, standing at the kitchen in my parents' home, my body caved in, and I found I was unable to do another thing. I stood, stunned, not knowing what to do; my whole body had seized up. It was a panic attack, although at the time I didn't recognise it as such. There was no one to turn to, certainly talking to anyone in my family was not an option. But I knew I could not keep going like this; I had to do something.

When the attack passed, secretly later that day I went to see the family doctor who lived down the road. I got the impression he was very aware of the whole situation. I wonder now if my mother used to confide in him about what was happening to me. She wouldn't have had any friends or family with whom to talk to about the circumstances of her life, but I imagine she possibly did spill to this family GP about my father's drinking, and her own problems. He suggested he make an appointment for me with a psychiatrist he highly recommended, whom he described as 'an approachable man'.

I can still see myself standing outside the grim, antiquated building of St Joseph's Hospital, formerly known as the Limerick Asylum. Built in 1827, like most of these places it was a structure that seemed designed to intimidate. I was petrified, but I forced my legs to keep moving down a cold, clinical corridor until I reached the psychiatrist's office.

I could barely breathe.

When I knocked and entered the room, he was sitting behind his desk, writing in his file, head down. He invited me to sit down. I sat at the edge of the chair in silence, unable to move. When he finished writing, he asked, 'Why are you here?' I did my best to explain. He began to soften slightly, and then decided the building wasn't suitable for us to meet, telling me, 'Breda I want to see you, but this is no place for me to see you.' He recommended a two-week stay in Milford House, a care centre in Castletroy, Limerick. There, he'd be able to see me as a private patient.

The relationship between my parents and me at that time was non-existent beyond mechanical exchanges about the running of the shop, looking after the smaller children or cooking meals, I just told them the doctor had advised me to go to Milford House for two weeks, and that was it.

I enjoyed my stay there. It was a kind of convalescent centre, not a psychiatric hospital.

The weather was sunny, and the grounds beautiful. I had the time of my life for two glorious weeks. I was free to come and go as I liked. No one treated me as if I had a mental illness. I cannot recall conversations with the psychiatrist, but I felt at ease with him. A medical report from St John of God Hospital, Dublin, states that he treated me 'for reactive depression with Valium only'.

Reactive depression and 'endogenous' depression were popular terms in the 1970s and 1980s. They were used to describe two kinds of depression – reactive being a reaction to distressing life events – while endogenous referred to depression resulting from internal biological factors such as chemical imbalances in brain chemistry.

At various stages I was diagnosed with having 'reactive depression'. Other times as suffering from 'endogenous depression'. In my case, psychiatry got it wrong. I never suffered from a chemical imbalance in my brain.

I like the term reactive depression because it makes sense of all I lived through. I wouldn't have been normal if I didn't feel gutted over the various things that happened to me.

Who wouldn't feel down when the home environment was so tense and unpredictable? I was constantly living in fear. One false move and there could be war. Who wouldn't feel down seeing their father heading to the pub every chance he got and coming home drunk? Who wouldn't feel down listening to the hot-headed rows that frequently erupted between my parents?

I was constantly on guard like a meek little mouse trying to make sure I kept myself safe. One wrong word or move could cause an uproar and either parent could end up giving out stink to me.

When I returned home, I was still unaware that driving myself to exhaustion was detrimental to my health or that there would be long-term consequences. The only way I knew to cope with life was to keep going and stay busy. I failed to notice that I was slowly undoing whatever benefits I'd gained from Milford House.

By the time my wedding day arrived, I was mentally and physically exhausted. I could hardly put one foot in front of the other when I tried to get out of bed that morning. My head felt weird; both temples throbbed with pain, and my body felt numb. I stood in front of the tall mirror in the hotel bedroom and struggled to put on my wedding dress. I was about to make a lifelong commitment to one particular man. What if I was wrong? And what about my health? I closed my eyes and stood motionless in the room. Intense, fast-moving, swirling sensations overwhelming me.

It made sense not to go ahead with the wedding; waiting for a few weeks was far better. Tommy would understand. But what about the guests who had travelled long distances to be there? I could imagine their shocked reactions and the resulting gossip. I didn't want to embarrass anyone, especially not Tommy. I had to go through with it.

There was knock on the bedroom door. My two sisters excitedly rushed into the room with a hairdresser and beautician. I was the centre of attention, with everyone fussing over me. I felt uncomfortable sitting in the chair, but I suppressed the swirling emotions and buried them deep inside me. When the beauticians finished their work, we made our way downstairs. The number of people gathered in the lobby took me by surprise. Their exuberant clapping and happy, beaming faces lifted me. I smiled back.

The wedding car was waiting outside. As the chauffeur opened the door, I looked at my dad in the back seat and was delighted to see him smiling and in good form. As the entourage made it to the church, I did my best to talk to him naturally, and he chatted back to me, but I can't remember what we said.

My youngest brother, who was a page boy, led the procession. My two sisters, the bridesmaids, followed. I felt a strong sense of relief as we approached the altar. Tommy had moved out from the pew to join me. I felt safe. My dad moved aside, and my eldest sister lifted the veil covering my face.

I wanted to enjoy the ceremony, but I felt too unwell. I glanced at Tommy kneeling beside me and wondered what he'd think if he could see how bad I felt. My body felt stiff and heavy. I barely remember our wedding vows, the exchange of rings, and the loud applause when the celebrant addressed Tommy and said, 'You may now kiss the bride.' Years later, he told me he knew how sick I was that day. I can't help thinking how incredible he was that he still went ahead with the wedding; not every man would.

Being the person in a marriage who is unwell in the way I was, you know the affect you're having on the people around you. It's a huge weight to carry. The guilt – you're so weighed down by it. All you want is to be well. To be yourself. You're doing everything in your power to make that happen, to get well again, and you're just getting worse and worse. It's the worst kind of despair. But it's hidden, because you don't know how to talk about it with your partner.

I would still have difficulties sharing a lot of stuff with Tommy about me as a person, things that I could share with my psychologist. Sometimes, if your partner hasn't had the experience of what you've lived through, then it's very hard to communicate with them. It's easier to talk to therapists. They have more of an intellectual understanding of what people can go through. Whereas Tommy had never met anyone depressed in his life before.

When Mass was over, the photographer moved to the front of the altar and took photos of the wedding party. The endless repetition of false smiles got to me.

Our wedding album shows a photo of Tommy kissing me in the back seat of the car before we set off for the hotel. Despite my ill health, I can't believe how happy I look in the photos. The chauffeur drove us to Teach Furbo Hotel, Spiddal, outside Galway city. Streamers adorned the cars, and the hooters sounded for the entire journey. I was amazed at the beautiful compliments and the number of people who wanted only the best for us. I had never experienced that before.

That evening, I was distraught when I caught sight of a large cohort of people around the bar. My dad's relationship with alcohol had a horrendous impact on our family. I was relieved that we could leave soon for Dublin Airport to catch the flight to Majorca, Spain, where we would spend two weeks on our honeymoon.

I had one more duty to perform. The single ladies gathered in the lobby. I walked forward, turned and threw my wedding bouquet over my shoulder.

I had never been on a plane before. Unfortunately, we hit severe turbulence that lasted most of the flight. Scared and unwell, I grasped Tommy's arm. Finally, the aircraft began its descent and wobbled to a grinding halt. We had arrived safely at Palma de Mallorca Airport.

Distressing feelings in my body stayed with me as we made our way to the taxi rank. The driver took us to Peguera, where we were booked into a hotel in the town centre. The porter met us at reception and brought us to our room. When he opened the door, we saw twin beds. I couldn't believe it – not on our wedding night!

I nudged Tommy and asked if we could have a different room. He said to the porter, 'Please, any chance of a room with a double bed?' He was told, 'All the rooms are similar because of the hot climate.' When he was gone, we shoved the beds together, unaware that because of the shiny tiled floor, they would keep slipping apart during the night.

I felt apprehensive that night but not in a scary way. Tommy and I had been courting for two years. I felt safe with him and loved, and I was looking forward to our first night together. During the days that followed, even though I was unwell throughout, a series of distractions made it easy to forget how I felt.

Palmira Beach, one of the most significant strands in the district, which lies beyond a beautiful promenade lined with palm trees, was just across the road. Next, we took a day trip by coach to Porto Cristo, a small, picturesque fishing village on the east coast of Majorca, where we visited a safari zoo.

We visited Cuevas del Drach (Caves of Drach), one of the island's main tourist attractions. The Baths of Diana had breathtaking waterfalls and cascades. Day trips and the sheer beauty of the place kept me going.

While the highs were exceptional, the lows I experienced in myself were painful. I was constantly uneasy and on edge but hid it well. We were newly married. Now more than ever, I wanted to keep up the pretence that I was okay. But it hurt that I couldn't be more open with Tommy.

Chapter 8

THE NURSE WHO RISKED EVERYTHING

We returned home in August 1973. We would be living in Connemara, in a home Tommy was building on land right beside the house he had grown up in, near Clifden. Our new bungalow wasn't finished, so we moved in with his parents, who welcomed us with open arms.

I tried to fit in but felt out of place. Now 23, I battled daily to rise above debilitating feelings and sensations but felt ill at ease. Like what a bad flu does to your body, I would have found it very hard to put one foot in front of the other. You're forcing your body to move when it doesn't want to. I struggled to find the words to explain why I felt as badly as I did. Not being able to express myself made conversations with my mother-in-law very difficult. My uneasy and complicated relationship with my own mother also contributed to the strain between us.

In mid-September, I was asked to play the organ for a local wedding. When I woke that Saturday morning, I couldn't move. No matter how hard I tried, I couldn't get out of bed. Eventually, I managed to manoeuvre myself off the mattress and made it as far as the farmhouse kitchen. I tried to make my way out to the back kitchen, the newer extension, but couldn't. Instead, I sat down beside the fire, Tommy's mother and father were coming in and out of the room; the very last people I would have wanted to see me in that state. There wasn't a hope of being able to play for the wedding, even the smallest effort felt almost beyond me. I became fixated on how I was letting the bride and groom down. Looking at the floor, I started to visibly shake all over. My instincts were to run out of the room, I desperately wanted to appear normal, but I couldn't move. Tommy and his parents witnessed all of this. I was mortified.

This was the first time Tommy had seen me have a panic attack up close. He phoned the local GP, who arrived at the house. I believed my poor health was primarily physical, so I agreed to be admitted to what was then Calvary General Hospital, in Galway. They were best positioned to diagnose the cause of my health problems. I was hopeful they would find out what was wrong with me. I genuinely thought it was an ordinary physical ailment.

Admission would also give Tommy a reasonable explanation to offer the bride and groom for my absence.

The usual tests were done, but my world fell apart again when all the results returned as normal. I went blank, with no idea of what was going to happen next. When the medical staff came near, I wondered if they viewed me suspiciously. Did the nurses think I was making it up and wasting everyone's time?

I understand now that to get out of the stressful situation, I had begun to dissociate, withdraw totally into a trance-like state in order to protect myself. It was similar to what had happened during the ECT treatments. Lying in the bed now, this is what I began to do.

Quite still, with my eyes closed, little did I know that arrangements were being made to transfer me to St Brigid's Hospital, the mental hospital in Ballinasloe, for what would be my second admission there. I opened them when I felt movement, to see

I was being lifted on a mattress into an ambulance without knowing where I was going.

A medical report noted:

> Shortly after her honeymoon, she was admitted to Calvary Hospital, Galway, where she remained in a trance or fit condition all day. She was transferred to St Brigid's Hospital, Ballinasloe, where she also remained in a trance or fit-like condition.

In the book *What Happened to You?* (co-authored by Oprah Winfrey), the writing of Dr Bruce D. Perry helped me to make sense of my reactions at that time:

> In the face of unavoidable pain and distress, a natural human response is to 'dissociate'.* The capacity to control your dissociative capabilities is very powerful ... It's one of your superpowers.†

I dissociated to avoid contact with the outside world. I lay in bed for days, oblivious to my surroundings; keeping this trance-like state going was the only way I could cope. I was aware I was doing it; from the outside, I was still, eyes closed, but I was alert inside.

After a couple of weeks I was discharged. Tommy had been

---

* Perry, Bruce, and Oprah Winfrey. *What Happened to You? Conversations on Trauma, Resilience and Healing.* S.L., Bluebird, 2021, p.280.
† Ibid, p.177.

fighting to get me out, ringing the hospital from the public phone box in our local village, asking was there any chance of getting me home.

I was relieved when he told me we no longer had to live with his parents and could move into our new home, which he had built. At the time, we had one bedroom, and one room to live in. Our kitchen table was made out of two barrels with a door placed across them.

Tommy had gone to England when he was 16, to his older brother, where he had trained as a carpenter. A few years before he met me, his mother wrote to her older son and mentioned how nice it would be if Tommy came home now that they were getting older. Tommy wasn't meant to see the letter, but he accidentally came across it. The minute he read it, he dropped everything and came home. Only for that, we would never have met. When he returned to Connemara, he started to build houses.

In those early years of married life, I continued to feel unable to share fully with him what I was experiencing; instead, I became more and more isolated and felt greater guilt and shame. To cope, I kept myself busy. I painted walls and made full-length Connemara tweed curtains for the front room.

One day, Tommy suggested that I learn to drive. Where we live is beautiful, but remote, so you need a car to get around. With great patience, he taught me the basics and gave me a few lessons in his car, after which I took the driving test and passed. He then surprised me with a second-hand Green Fiat 500 that he bought for me so that I would no longer be confined to the house.

I was able to accept an offer of work as a music teacher in the local primary schools. This involved teaching a variety of instruments to individual students and forming a school band and choir.

Our new bungalow was coming along nicely. One Saturday morning, as we drove to Galway to pick up some furniture, we were blinded by the sun and hit a mound of gravel on the verge of the road. I hit my head on the dashboard as Tommy jammed on the brakes. We managed to get out of the car, and before we knew where we were, a crowd of people had gathered to help. I was encouraged to see the local GP, who ensured I was okay. The furniture money we'd saved had to be spent repairing the car. In the meantime Tommy needed the Green Fiat 500 to get to work. Without my own transport, I couldn't get to the schools to teach.

Stuck at home, I managed as best I could, but soon became lost in my own dark, isolated inner world and made no attempts to relate to anyone. My mood levels dropped to an unprecedented low. Eventually, our GP referred me to the Psychiatric Unit in Galway.

When we arrived, the receptionist said, 'I'm sorry, but you'll have to return home and come back again tomorrow. We have no beds.' When I asked to see a psychiatrist, she replied, 'There's no one available.' When Tommy intervened, he got no satisfaction. He went in search of a men's room before facing into the drive home.

As I sat waiting for him, doing my utmost to appear normal, I wondered if there was a way to convince the authorities that I needed help, and began to feel scared I wouldn't be able to get it, and instead would be sent back on the 60-mile drive home. Panicked, my body started to shake in violent spasms, and my head felt as if it might explode. I was having a panic attack. Two male nurses in white uniforms dashed forward. One put me lying on the floor and jammed me underneath his body. I tried to fight him off, but that was impossible. His colleague injected me intravenously with Nembutal. A few minutes later, I was forced into a straitjacket. A doctor signed a detention order. The medical form read, 'Family unavailable.' No one checked the bathroom. I was taken by ambulance to St Brigid's Hospital, Ballinasloe for the third time. It was 38 miles away, and I was transferred against my will and without Tommy's knowing.

On arrival at St Brigid's institution, my condition was described as 'Quite heavily sedated ... conversation all mixed up, impossible to make any sense of it.' The following day, when Tommy and my parents came to bring me to the Psychiatric Unit in Galway, they were only allowed to see the doctor and were refused permission to go anywhere near me. I wasn't told at any stage that they had come to collect me.

> **File notes:** St Brigid's Hospital, 28/10/73. I interviewed this lady's husband and her father and mother. I understand from them that she attended here as an extern for ECT some time ago. They also say that she was treated in Dublin, where she also had ECT. She has since been treated by the family doctor, who has told them that the ECT should not have been given to her. And that she has been treated wrongly both here and in Dublin!

Copies of my hospital chart, which I recently managed to retrieve through GDPR, state that I suffered from 'hysterical seizures', that I was 'impossible to control', and repeatedly tried 'to get out of bed'. My memory is of deliberately resisting when the nurses tried to inject me forcefully and on one occasion getting out of bed to walk around to calm myself and stay in touch with reality.

My efforts to resist what I experienced as coercive and brutal control resulted in my being forced into a straitjacket and strapped into a bed with iron rails on both sides. I was restrained for the next 11 days and only allowed to use a commode at set times, under supervision.

One report from St Brigid's Hospital dated 29 October 1973 states that I was treated for epilepsy with 'Gardenal grs [grammes] TDS and Mysoline 250mg', despite another doctor's insistence that my seizures were 'a hysterical phenomenon'. In addition, I was prescribed 'Sodium Amytal grs three orally at night and repeat' and 'Nembutal grs, 4 plus 50mgs Largactil, intramuscular.'

> **File notes:** 30-10-73. ... in a car accident some weeks ago. (She) probably had a head injury and may be heading for grand-mal epilepsy. History of concussion. Intelligent, it seems to me. She had to be sedated again this morning as she refused oral medication.

How hitting my head off the dashboard during a minor car crash ended up in a psychiatric report as a 'history of concussion' still baffles me.

Two nurses took me out of the straitjacket early one afternoon, and one brought me by wheelchair to the day room. I was shocked by the sight of countless elderly patients sitting side by side on chairs, in a vegetative state, motionless and unresponsive. I couldn't see precisely how many patients there were as the room stretched further than I could see.

I didn't dare object, although my whole body wanted to scream 'No!' to how we were being treated. Later that evening, I was wheeled back to the ward. On the way, I began to fear that if I didn't get out soon, I could be there for the rest of my life. There was no access to phones in these hospitals, so I was never able to contact Tommy, my one source of sanctuary. We didn't have a phone in our house, the only phone at the time was a public one in Cleggan village nearby. He would have to go down to the village to ring to see how I was doing, and if I had been moved, would only find out then. I believe he was the one responsible for getting me home each time, by repeatedly calling and asking.

This was the reason that I asked the nurse one night in November, as I lay in the ward trapped in a straitjacket to ring my parents. Their phone was in the shop, I knew it was more likely she would be able to reach them than Tommy.

'I can't do that; I'll lose my job if I do that.' She sounded genuinely terrified.

It felt hopeless.

Soon after that encounter, possibly the next morning, I heard my father's voice coming from nearby. I wondered if I was imagining it. He was shouting, raising quite a storm. I listened to what sounded like a heated argument. He was here. Very close by. I hadn't been forgotten. The nurse had risked everything to help me.

Someone raised their voice to my father. 'She's a danger to society and cannot be discharged,' I heard them say. This made no sense at all, given I felt completely powerless.

My father raised his voice even more. 'I don't care what you say. I will not allow anyone to treat my daughter like this.' His voice grew even louder as he walked towards me. Looking in at me, he removed the steel rails around the bed, undid the straps, and released me from the straitjacket. Bending over, he lifted me into his arms and carried me down the corridor, ignoring the protests of the staff. He didn't stop until he had me safely outside the main door.

Tommy was waiting in our car. I was too sick to relate to him. My body was limp, floppy and barely conscious. I needed assistance to be placed in the back seat beside him. Dad drove straight to Dublin. With the help of my parents' GP in Limerick, arrangements had been made with St Vincent's Hospital, Elm Park, Dublin, to have me admitted. I was 23. Everything changed when I got there.

Chapter 9

THANK YOU FOR HEARING ME

Two days after admission to St Vincent's psychiatric unit, I was sitting on the edge of a chair waiting for breakfast to be served. I still felt awful and could hardly move, but at least my surroundings had improved. At the time, Vincent's was a brand-new psychiatric unit. It was light, and lovely; I remember thinking this is like going from hell to heaven.

I was in a fairly bad state, feeling as if there was no hope for me. I could barely move. I was weaker than ever before in my life. I was in too intense a numbed state to put any words on what I was going through. I was stiff like a poker.

All I could do was hang on and endure each moment as I sat there motionless on the chair in the corridor waiting for everyone to be called in to the dining room for breakfast. Not knowing what was going to happen to me next was petrifying. I was at the mercy of others. I had no control whatsoever over the way my life was going. I was lucid, I was in touch with the reality of my situation, but I felt as if the whole world was against me.

I had to hope against hope I was now in a safe place and that against the odds a way would be found to improve both my mental and physical health. I feared I was just another patient sitting in a row of chairs that nobody was taking any notice of.

I noticed a man coming towards me, it was the medical director. At the time, I just knew him as the man in charge. I didn't think he could actually be coming to speak to me, so I just kept the head down, but he knelt beside me on one knee, placed his hand on my right shoulder, and said in a warm, kind voice, 'Breda, I know you're feeling unwell. But I am hoping that you'll be able to do something for me today.' Hearing those words when you are at your lowest is startling. He continued speaking; 'There's an important conference taking place in the hospital. Doctors and psychiatrists from all over Ireland and abroad will be in attendance. If you could find it in yourself to go in to those people and tell them what has reduced you to this appalling state of health – and it's quite okay if you don't feel up to it – but I'm hopeful that in the future, what you have to say will have a real impact on the way doctors treat their patients. Many people could be spared the terrible suffering you've had to endure. You would be making a big difference. What do you think?'

I considered my options and agreed. One thing I hated in those institutions was boredom, I couldn't stand trying to pass the time with nothing to do. Cruel boredom, it ate into my soul. This would pass the time and I had absolutely nothing to lose. I couldn't feel worse than I already did. From feeling powerless and useless to anyone, perhaps this was a chance to make a real difference.

A couple of hours later, I sat waiting in a busy corridor for the director to arrive. I felt apprehensive but calm. He greeted me with a warm smile. I was weak but managed to stand up. He asked if I was okay, and I assured him I was. I had nothing prepared, but if I say yes to something, I do it.

Linking my arm, he led me into a large hall and escorted me to a podium. Vincent's felt different to the other psychiatric hospitals I spent time in; you were treated with respect and dignity. I held on to the rail and climbed a couple of steps; my legs were wobbling; I was as weak as water. When I reached the stand, I grasped the wooden surround tightly to stop myself from falling.

Looking out into the auditorium, I saw a large gathering of people in tiered seating arranged in a semi-circle. The room was packed, and they were all looking right at me. I wasn't sure what to say or what they expected of me. For a moment, I felt panic, but then I decided that the easiest thing to do would be to start with my childhood.

After a shaky start, my words flowed effortlessly, perhaps due to the sheer relief of having people listen to me without interrupting. Or maybe my confidence grew as I felt they understood. There was silence in the room. After describing my childhood, I spoke about what had happened to me in St Patrick's Hospital, Dublin, the psychiatric unit, Galway and St Brigid's Hospital, Ballinasloe. You could have heard a pin drop in that room, it was incredible. I don't know where it came from, but I'm so proud I got to say all of it. I ended with the words, 'I'm convinced that bad experiences can wreck a person's health just as much as any serious illness.'

The audience rose to their feet and applauded. I was very surprised and somewhat puzzled. I've never had that response to me as a person. I could feel the support in the room. Overwhelmed, I thought, *Get me out of here*, and stumbled as I tried to make my way down from the podium to leave. Immediately, the medical director rushed to my assistance and linked my arm to lead me out. I felt he understood: *There is more to her story than meets the eye.* He was radically different to any other psychiatrist whose care I was under. The audience was still clapping hard. That they thought well of me gave me new courage. They made me want to get well. I promised myself I would.

Over the next few days in St Vincent's, I did begin to improve. I met with a female psychiatrist whom I liked. In September 2022, I was surprised to see in my medical records that what I regarded as ordinary conversations with her were classified as psychotherapy. I also see from my file that I attended group therapy sessions, but I don't remember being there. I didn't realise at the time that this was therapy – it didn't feel like it was going anywhere, that there was a plan, which is I think why talking didn't help at this point.

The doctors, nurses, and staff I met at St Vincent's psychiatric hospital couldn't have been more helpful, their approach felt different from what I had experienced in other hospitals. My only disappointment was that there was little to do between meetings and mealtimes. I needed to be involved in some activity, preferably something that would challenge my mind.

Eventually, I mustered the courage to ask permission to walk around the grounds.

Not only was I given permission to walk around the grounds, but they said it was fine to take a bus to the nearest shopping centre. That I was trusted was a great boost to my self-esteem.

I took a bus and meandered around the shops. There was a buzz in the air. I had to readjust quickly to an environment so different from the hospital wards I'd just come from. I bought some new clothes to look my best when I returned home. When I noticed myself beginning to feel weak, I headed straight back to the hospital.

Two days later, the boredom got to me again. I asked the nurse at reception if I could be discharged. She discussed my request with my doctor, and their reply was that they'd prefer me to stay. But on Sunday, 25 November, I signed myself out. They respected my decision.

> **Discharge summary:** 28 November '73. During her stay in the psychiatric unit, Breda was treated with group and individual psychotherapy in which her symptoms were discussed in depth and the psychological implications were examined. On this regime, she did reasonably well and had no panic attacks during her stay in the hospital. She showed a certain amount of insight into the psychological factors associated with her panic attacks. However, after two weeks in the hospital, Breda refused to remain any longer in spite of our encouragement to continue to work on her problems.
>
> Interestingly, during her stay in the Unit, Breda did not exhibit any symptoms of depression. She ate and slept normally, and her only medication was 5mgs Valium at night. We regret that Breda did not remain longer in the Unit since two weeks was hardly sufficient to consolidate her improvement. We hope that she continues to do well.

Remarkably, the psychiatrist did not prescribe heavy drugs – 'only medication was 5mgs Valium at night.' My experience there was of feeling respected and listened to, rather than misdiagnosed, restrained and drugged against my will in St Brigid's Hospital, Ballinasloe.

Chapter 10

A MOTHER KNOWS

My experience of childbirth has taught me that a mother knows best what's happening in her body. Had I been listened to, and my words taken seriously and acted upon, my first baby's life could have been saved. I want to share what I learned through losing my son, Dermot, if only to make his three days on this earth count for something.

I was delighted when I found out I was pregnant. Despite debilitating nausea, I kept going every day. Instead of taking things easy, I drove myself hard to stay on top of household chores. As well as feeling physically sick, I was sick in myself.

I was afraid that if I tried to explain how difficult I found each day, people wouldn't understand. They might interpret my discomfort and distress as mental illness. Thankfully, life became easier for me after the first four months of my pregnancy, as the sickness eased off slightly.

At Easter, Tommy and I travelled to Limerick to spend time with my family, as we always did at Christmas and occasionally at the weekend. As a younger teenager, the odd time we would go north with my family to visit my father's side, but watching my father get more and more drunk as we stopped at pubs took away the enjoyment for me. This day though is a lovely memory to look back on. On Bank Holiday Monday, we all, including Daddy, headed out to a beautiful hamlet in Portroe, County Tipperary, and it was really nice.

In glorious sunshine, we had a lovely family picnic. I was

five months pregnant, and I couldn't have been happier. I was looking forward to that little baby so much.

Life continued as usual, and the months flew by after we came home. I was becoming more excited by the day. The baby was due on 31 July 1974, the day after our wedding anniversary. My gynaecologist assured me all was well.

That August, I was admitted to the maternity unit. I was 10 days overdue, and nothing was happening. This was my first baby, and I didn't know what to expect but trusted that I was safe. Lying on the flat of my back in bed, nothing happened for several hours. By nightfall, I was becoming very anxious. At 2 a.m., I found the courage to speak out and tell a passing nurse I was worried. She replied, 'It's your first baby. You could be in labour for a long time. There's nothing unusual about that!'

When she returned, I was agitated and begged her to get the gynaecologist. I had a strong sense that something wasn't right. I had been far too long in labour with nothing happening. She ignored me. Later, I was led to believe that nurses were too afraid to call private consultants during the middle of the night unless necessary. No one realised the baby and I were in danger.

At 4.10 a.m., another nurse checked how much I had dilated. I could tell from the expression on her face that something was seriously wrong. She rushed away. Within minutes, I was wheeled into the delivery ward. The gynaecologist arrived, and without wasting a second, he assisted me.

I drifted in and out of consciousness. I asked the nurse if my husband could come in. She checked with the gynaecologist. He shouted at her, 'I've enough to do to try and keep this mother and baby alive. No!'

What happened was terrifying. It was as if my body was taken over by an intense blackness. I could see it happen but could do nothing about it. I was convinced I was going to die. I heard a voice say that my blood pressure was dangerously high.

The gynaecologist called for forceps. Finally, my baby was born. I overheard that it was a little boy. There was a commotion in the room when I opened my eyes. A nurse brushed past me with the baby in her arms. I was wheeled to a private room without a word.

After what felt like a very long time, I was informed that my baby was in the premature baby unit (PBU). However, I wasn't allowed to see him. In a very dismissive, offhand way, the staff nurse told me that he was suffering from hydrocephalus and spina bifida.

The following morning, another nurse rushed in. She couldn't get her words out fast enough. 'I'm sorry, but your baby is not expected to live. I need your permission to have him baptised by the hospital chaplain.' I was stunned. Moving from foot to foot, notebook in hand, she asked, 'What's the baby's name?' Terror-stricken, the words stuck in my throat. Somehow, I managed to say, 'Dermot Thomas'. She dashed out of the room.

A meeting with the gynaecologist for Tommy and I was arranged. I was in a terrible state but made it down the corridor to the room where he was waiting. Hearing the tragic news again from him, a professional, struck me with an added blow.

After that, all I can recall is being back in bed alone and becoming more agitated by the minute. Overpowered, I cried loudly and pulled the bed covers over my head to hide from the world. Years later, reading *The Choice* by Edith Eger, I recognised myself in her words: '(When) we are overwhelmed by loss (we) think that we will never recover a sense of self and purpose, that we will never mend.'*

The next day, I insisted on seeing my baby. Tommy helped me out of the bed. I held his arm, and we slowly walked down the corridor to the PBU. When we got there, the nurse refused us entry. In an unfeeling way, she said, 'You can only look through the small pane of glass over there. When you do, I'll point out the incubator to you.'

I stretched up on my toes as far as I could to try and get a glimpse of Dermot's face. I saw the outline of his head. I clamped up. I was too afraid of authority to stand up to them and demand to see more of him. All we could do was return to the ward. Neither Tommy nor I said a word.

The following morning, 11 August 1973, the gynaecologist broke the news that Dermot had died. I heard babies in a nearby ward crying alone. That tore me apart. On trips to the bathroom, I met mothers carrying their newborn infants. My baby was dead. I couldn't take any more.

I asked to be allowed home. A nurse told me the doctor wouldn't hear of it. But I knew I couldn't stay there. I discharged myself. Tommy and his sister came to pick me up. They helped me into the front passenger seat. I didn't say a word. I was in agony.

We headed to the local hospital, where I was admitted. The next day, I was too unwell to attend Dermot's funeral. A visitor

---

* Eger, Edith Eva. *The Choice*. London, Rider, 2018, p.234.

from our parish told me that Tommy had carried the tiny white coffin up the church aisle alone. By the end of the week, I was allowed home from the hospital with a prescription for Valium.

Fifty years later, that image of Tommy and the memory of not being able to be there for him is still painful. I regret that I never got to hold my baby in my arms or see him laid out after he died.

Why couldn't I hold him close, not even during his last hours on earth? Why wasn't I allowed to touch him at any stage during the three days after his birth? Perhaps that was hospital policy then, but those rules left me with a chronic grief I've never been able to resolve.

We returned to meet the gynaecologist to hear the post-mortem results. We attended his private rooms where he welcomed both of us and expressed his heartfelt sympathy for the death of our baby. He invited us to sit down, and in a kind, gentle, compassionate way, he said, 'You will be relieved to hear that the post-mortem results show you had a perfectly healthy baby.'

He continued: 'I accept full responsibility for the death of your baby. You would have had a caesarean section if I had been there. When I arrived, it was too late. Your baby had moved too far down the birth canal. It was because you were ten days overdue that the baby's head had moulded. The whole effort of being born the usual way was too hard on his heart. I'm sorry.'

His honesty was uncompromising. He didn't hold back. Every word rang true. That didn't take away our grief, but it helped bring closure. I admired the gynaecologist's honesty and remained under his care for the rest of my pregnancies.

Dermot's short life highlights the need for maternity staff to listen to what mothers in labour say and take it seriously. And where there is loss, to ensure proper care for traumatised and bereaved women. Finally, his death reminds medical staff that kindness and honesty are the best responses to such tragedies.

I still can't go near Dermot's grave. Occasionally, I sense his presence close to me, especially when I open up and chat with him. Without fail, every year, I do this on his birthday. The late John O'Donoghue, Irish poet, said that our loved ones who have passed are but a thin veil away.

> The dead are not distant or absent. They are alongside us. When we lose someone to death, we lose their physical image and presence; they slip out of visible form into invisible presence. This alteration of form is the reason we cannot see the dead. But because we cannot see them does not mean they are not there.*

---

* O'Donohue, John. *Divine Beauty: The Invisible Embrace*. London; New York, Bantam Press, 2004, p.223.

Chapter 11

GIVING SORROW WORDS

It's difficult for those who've never struggled with mental health issues to appreciate how long it takes to recover. I would love to be able to say I walked away from St Vincent's Hospital – where people had listened very respectfully to what I needed to say – in late 1973 and left the trauma of my past behind me. But it doesn't work like that. Deep wounds take time to heal. We need not just one but repeated experiences of being heard and accepted with a person we trust who makes us feel safe. We need people who can help us make sense of why we feel and behave as badly as we do.

A month after Dermot died, I returned to teaching in the local community school. At the time, I was reliant on Valium tranquillisers. His death weighed heavily on my mind. I had feelings of grief and pent-up anger that I did not know how to resolve.

I hadn't the words to share my grief with Tommy. Neither of us spoke about Dermot. We just kept trying to get through each day as best we could.

As Halloween approached, I wondered about taking a child out of the orphanage for weekends. I asked Tommy, and he was all in favour. We went to see the nun in charge. She was friendly and polite, but I was stunned when she said, 'How do you feel about taking two instead of one? We have two young sisters who have been through a lot. Going to you at weekends would be great for them.' Tommy and I looked at one another as if to say, 'What do we do now?' We agreed to take both.

Arrangements were made for me to pick the girls up the following Friday evening on my way home from school. We got on well over the coming weeks, and they enjoyed their stay. I was delighted when the nun told me they had also been happier in the orphanage since they had started coming to us.

As we had planned to have them stay with us for Christmas, I asked them what they'd like from Santa. Immediately, they both exclaimed, 'A tricycle!' The truth was we couldn't afford them. But Tommy and I discussed the matter and decided we couldn't let the girls down.

We were all up bright and early on Christmas morning to see what Santa had left in the front room. The girls unwrapped their presents. When the younger one discovered her tricycle, she stood back in astonishment and began to jump up and down, saying, 'It's delicious like sweets. It's delicious like sweets.' I gazed at her face, radiant with joy. Then, she jumped up on the tricycle and took off down the hall with her bigger sister following her on her trike.

Throughout January, we continued to have them stay with us at weekends. Then, for some unknown reason, the older sister became sullen and moody and reacted badly whenever I tried to say something to her or asked her to do something small.

If only I had felt comfortable enough to approach her, ask her what was wrong, sit down with her, listen to what she had to say and try to get to the root of the problem. But it wasn't my place to pry into her family history when the superior in the orphanage hadn't put me in the picture.

Today, I wonder what her life was like before she ended up in an orphanage. What happened to her? Could the contrast between the love she experienced in our home and her experiences up to that time have been confusing?

I was also still struggling with my health, and her offhand behaviour dragged me down.

I tried to react lovingly and kindly, but that made no difference. I began to dread their visits. I wanted to back out, but the nun encouraged me to give it another try. 'The girls love going to you. You're making a big difference in their lives.' Despite intense reservations, I agreed to let them keep coming. I tolerated the situation for three weekends until I couldn't stand it any longer. I didn't know how to face the nun again and kept putting it off.

Then the phone rang one morning, and I heard her say the children had measles. I jumped at the opportunity and said, 'I'm sorry, but under the circumstances, I won't be able to take them anymore as I'm trying to get pregnant.' She understood.

We never saw the girls again. I was relieved for a while that I no longer had to worry about them, but as time passed, the more guilty I felt. Bad enough that the girls, for whatever reason, had been abandoned once without me causing that to happen to them a second time.

Tommy had no problem with either of the two sisters, so I wondered what it was about me that I was on edge with the older sibling. I wish things could have worked out differently for all of us.

In April 1975, I was delighted to be pregnant again. I had all the classic signs: nausea, weakness, and my tummy and breasts getting more prominent. There wasn't a question in my mind but that there was another baby on the way. I had been through the early stages of pregnancy before and didn't see any need for a check-up until some weeks later.

After routine checks, the doctor stood before his desk and said matter-of-factly, 'You're not pregnant.' I didn't believe him and insisted on a pregnancy test. The result came back negative. I was sure there had been some mistake. I returned home, still convinced I was pregnant.

A phantom pregnancy, also termed pseudocyesis, is the absolute belief that one is pregnant. According to researchers, most evidence shows that pseudocyesis is common in women who intensely desire to become pregnant or have lost a child. The intensity fires a signal to the brain and the rest of the body, gradually developing all the usual signs of pregnancy. Research has also shown that in some cases, a woman may have elevated levels of oestrogen or prolactin, which can give rise to physical symptoms combined with a strong desire to bond with a baby.

I needed help to process the impact of the phantom pregnancy on my mental health and wellbeing. There were no beds available in the Galway Psychiatric Unit. In May 1975, the GP arranged for me to be admitted to St John of God psychiatric hospital in Dublin. I wasn't happy with this, but I recognised I had to do something. It was my first time staying there.

When we got to Dublin, we had some hours to kill before checking in to the hospital, and Tommy suggested we go to Powerscourt, in Wicklow. I was really unwell by now, hardly able to put one foot in front of the other; my general wellbeing at the time was at such a low ebb my ability to function was impacted and I was barely ticking over, but the beauty of that place, being out in nature, was gorgeous.

The time came to go, and I was as nervous as a bag of cats, intimidated and wondering what was going to happen to me. But still, hoping for the best, I thought maybe here I would find the help I needed. Maybe I would find a way, with the right help.

After completing the usual admission procedures, a nurse appeared. 'Come with me,' she said, and escorted us to St Anne's ward on the third floor. I will never forget that place. Of every place I have been admitted to, this was the worst, apart from St Brigid's in Ballinasloe. Tommy and I mechanically followed her down a corridor, doors we passed through locking behind us.

She passed us over to another nurse, who showed me to a small room, accessed through more locked doors. I didn't know then it was an isolation room. Tommy was still with me for now. The room was bare except for a single bed, jammed up against the bare white wall beside the door and a small window lined with bars running from end to end. There was no chair to sit on, so Tommy sat at the bottom of the bed. I asked him, 'Please will you try and find a shop where you can get me a paint-by-numbers kit?' He had to knock on the door to be let out. When he left, the door was locked again, and I felt very alone.

Apart from my pyjamas, my clothes, money and jewellery were taken from me, and I was ordered into bed, between the starched white sheets. I was in a state of shock. You lie there, trying to survive, trying not to burst into tears.

There was a knock at the door, and it was Tommy. He was told he could only stay a few minutes more. He was probably as distraught as I was. But what can you do? What could we even say to one another? I was hanging on to his presence like an anchor. I needed the paint-by-numbers kit for my sanity, because what would I do when Tommy had gone?

As soon as the door slammed behind him it was locked again. Frantically, I took the various components out of the box and began to paint. If I hadn't had that, I would have gone insane. It gave me something to occupy my mind. My freedom had been totally taken away from me. I wasn't that sick to warrant this. It was cruel.

The next morning, the door was unlocked, and I was led down to breakfast.

Against my will, I was kept in that isolation room on St Anne's ward for three days and three nights.

Every morning after breakfast, patients were allowed to sit for a while on a line of chairs in a dark, gloomy narrow passage with doors off it. I don't know if it was all isolation rooms. Those I met in the corridor were heavily medicated and looked as if they were living in a different world. I felt on edge on that ward, yet the doctor's note in my file, dated 26 May, reads: 'Patient quite happily settled in hospital. Not overly depressed.'

The one beautiful experience of being on St Anne's ward was that I met Maeve. A fellow patient, she was around the same age, and we had lots in common. As we sat side by side in that corridor and chatted quietly to one another, I began to come back to myself.

In hushed tones, so none of the staff would overhear, she told me I hadn't a hope of getting out of this place until they decided I was not a danger to the people around me, and that

I was mentally okay, but it was they who would decide that. To hear that was so frightening. Talk about having to be on your best behaviour. It felt like showing how you truly felt would result in being punished.

After sitting in the corridor for what felt like about half an hour, it was back to the isolation room for the rest of the day bar mealtimes.

Part of my mind has blotted out much of these stays, so difficult were they. Also, the ECTs severely affected my memory.

Two or three days later, they decided it was safe to let me down to St Joseph's ward, which was a much freer space and nicer environment.

I felt traumatised by what I witnessed in St Anne's ward at St John of God – to what patients had been reduced to: zombie-ish states, in a way more severe than anything I had seen elsewhere. Big, grown, hefty men, out of it. All these decades later, I still find it hard to think about it, because I don't believe any human being should be reduced to that. I feel I went to that hospital to get well and ended up traumatised beyond anything I had experienced previously, by what I saw, and how I was treated.

On the second floor, there was more freedom, but one still had to adhere strictly to the rules or suffer the consequences: a heavier drug prescription or being detained longer. Before admission to St John of God Hospital, I had been prescribed Valium 10mg three times a day and night and two Mogadon sleeping tablets for what staff described as my 'fainting attacks'.

During intensely emotional confrontations at home with Tommy, my world would become overwhelming, and I felt I had no control. I had learned to cope by dropping on the floor and appearing to faint. I closed my eyes or stared into space and went into a trance. That kind of dissociation not only stopped rows but gave me time to gather myself together. If there was a full-scale row going on between us, and it was hell for leather and I felt like I couldn't get through to him and he didn't understand where I was coming from, I would feel so afraid and unsafe, that I would panic and dissociate. It was really my body screaming, *I can't take any more of this. How do I get out of it?* It was very hard on Tommy, having to witness me like that. I remember feeling a certain satisfaction that Tommy could no longer give out to me or drive his point home because I was in too bad a state. Now I was the one in the driving seat, so to speak, and it put an end to the row. It's hard to admit all this, but it's the truth.

In St John of God Hospital, I couldn't risk expressing my anger after witnessing how patients were often treated harshly, especially on St Anne's ward. I relied on visits from Tommy to tell him what was happening. The only thing I had to hang onto was that he was coming up at the weekend. I wanted to tell him what I had seen up in St Anne's. There was no question of talking to any of the hospital staff about it, or about how I felt. The medication would be upped, and whatever hope I had of getting home would go out the window.

When he phoned Wednesday evening, a nurse told me to take the call in the hall. When I heard him say, 'Breda, I'm so sorry about this, but I won't be able to come up at the weekend.' I was gutted. I tried to convince him of how urgently I needed him to come, but he insisted he couldn't. I was desperate, lost my cool and abruptly put down the phone.

File notes: 29 May. Patient quite content in hospital. Not depressed. No 'attacks'. Had a row with her husband on the phone yesterday. He isn't coming up at the weekend. Rather hysterical reaction to this. I discussed this with her and pointed out how demanding and unreasonable she was in her reaction to him. May have a one-night pass at the weekend if husband comes. Valium 5mgs twice daily and night. Stop in a week.

I had started group therapy, although I have no recollection of being at those sessions. I only discovered that I did attend later when I read my file. A female psychiatrist spent time with me, asking about my past.

File notes: 5 June. I had a long interview with Mrs O' Toole this morning. She was quite tense and anxious at the beginning but relaxed and spoke frankly. Not overly depressed, eating and sleeping well. No 'fits' since admission. She is oversensitive and preoccupied with becoming pregnant again. Her weekend went quite well, but she was worried all the time, 'Is Tommy enjoying this place?' etc. Yesterday, she felt she was 'drifting'. Today, in much better form and more positive in her outlook.

The following evening, I chatted with a fellow patient, a priest. He listened intently and understood how hard I was finding the daily routine in the hospital. I felt safe with him, and believed he wouldn't betray my confidence. I told him what I had been too ashamed to say to anyone else until then. That I had always been conscious during my 'attacks' when I had pretended to faint. With his encouragement, I also confided this to my psychiatrist.

> **File notes:** 7 June. Mrs O'Toole was rather excited at first and told me that she had, for the first time, last night, confided to another patient that she did know what went on when she was in an 'attack'. She says that she felt great relief after doing so and, on his advice, decided to tell a nurse, me and another patient with whom she is friendly. She still has no idea why she kept up the pretence or why she had 16 attacks. She wonders if she should tell her husband. She maintains that their relationship is a good one, although he is inclined to be nervous 'in a different way'. The background should be more fully explored.

I recall leaving her office in tears after our sessions. I didn't know what to do with myself or where to turn. Talking about my early childhood took a lot out of me. My efforts seemed to get me nowhere. It felt like all I was doing was opening old wounds while the psychiatrist took notes. I kept my head down while uncomfortable sensations seared through my body.

At least on this occasion, some effort was made to explore those aspects of my life that had shaped the person I'd become, especially the death of our first baby and a phantom pregnancy. What seemed to be missing was any attempt to help me make links between my past and present so that I could make sense of my own behaviour and not feel so bad about myself. There was no plan.

Looking back, I wonder how different my stay might have

been if I had been taught some of the basic self-care skills I practise today. For example, we were never encouraged or shown how to practise meditation, or the importance of exercising daily, important ways I now manage my moods and catch myself, so I'm not so easily carried away by unpleasant thoughts. Connecting with nature, practising kindness to myself and others, being grateful, nurturing healthy life-affirming relationships, and living in the moment are also critical to my staying well.

The monotonous humdrum of each day in the hospital was cruel. I enjoyed the freedom of being out in the fresh air in nature and longed to wander around. But I was conscious of people watching my every step. That kind of supervision may have been comforting for some, but I found it insulting to my intelligence, trustworthiness and individuality.

Tommy was up that weekend, and I got the courage to tell him the truth about the fainting, and what had really been going on. He was so beautiful about it. He was taken aback, but once he comprehended what I was saying, he said 'Breda, it's not a problem, don't be worried about that, it's okay.' I felt very ashamed about my behaviour; I had been like a two-year-old child throwing a tantrum at times. But that was my dissociation.

> **File notes:** 9 June. A long interview with Mrs O' Toole. She seemed rather excited again. Told her husband everything – about her 'attacks' – he took it well and was very understanding. Her earliest recollection – as a child being thrown into her cot on a Sunday afternoon while her parents went to bed – being left there for hours – frightened and 'bored' to tears. She also remembers being

locked out in the garden with her younger brother as a child. She never got on with her mother. She recalls her mother taking her aside when she was about 12 and telling her something would happen to her soon, that she would bleed from the tops of her legs – this really confused her. She was ignorant of the facts of life until she was in her twenties.

She had a few hard experiences with males after she left the convent, which upset her. At the age of 19 years, on her first date, she went home with a boy, and he made a dive at her – she ran for her life. Two other similar experiences. Denies any sexual experiences in her childhood. Still sleeps poorly and complains of severe pre-menstrual tension. To see again in the morning.

Childhood very unhappy – very frightened of her father, a very heavy drinker, and of the frequent fights between her parents. Two mildly handicapped siblings – her sister had convulsions when she was younger – she remembers her having one at night. They shared the same bed. Another frightening experience. To continue Valium 2mg.'

File notes: 12 June. Long interview with Mrs O'Toole. Quite tense and upset. 'I'm not getting any better.'

On Friday, 20 June, a psychiatrist I hadn't seen before came and led me to a small consultation room. From her demeanour, I could tell she was courteous, respectful, and kind. After I sat on the chair in front of her desk, she said, 'Breda, I want to talk to you specifically about the death of your baby.'

I felt a surge of relief. At last, they were interested in the root of my poor health. During our conversation, I was open and honest. When the interview was over, there wasn't a doubt in my mind that other meetings would follow. Over the coming days, I waited and waited and waited to be called, but I never saw her again. That hit hard. Did those entrusted with my care not know I was grieving my baby?

> **File notes:** 16 June. Mrs O'Toole discussed her baby's death with me. It was clear that she has had a very unfortunate experience and that she blamed herself in part for it. She fears that she has caused the problem by not being certain about her 'dates' which may have influenced the decision to induce her and also feels guilty about being 'too unwell'. She fears that she will have problems with future pregnancies. She was told after the post-mortem that the child was not abnormal in any way.

My mother was contacted to arrange a family interview in St John of God. Initially, she was outraged and slammed down the phone after telling the doctor that my problems had nothing to do with them as I was married. Following intervention from Tommy, both my parents agreed to attend. Two family sessions took place the following weekend, one with Tommy and another with my parents and two of my siblings.

> **File notes:** 30 June. The patient was critical of both parents. Her siblings were also critical of their parents and thought they had little enjoyment of home life. Mother, in

particular, seems to expect unreasonably high standards of attainment and achievement from her children.

She seems preoccupied with the cost of everything. Children felt they were never allowed friends at home and were not trusted. This has led their behaviour to become deceitful and thus created a vicious circle. Their knowledge of their parents' early life was scant. Mother left home at 15 and went to England, not knowing why. Married at 25. Her husband is ten years older.

The patient's father drank heavily for many years, and the children all remembered rows, et cetera. Parents were badly off financially during the early years of marriage. The patient's main complaint about her parents was the heavy demands they made on her as a child. She also had to study hard and had no recreation. I pointed out to her that this seems to have been the general treatment of all her siblings, too. The second problem has been the lack of communication from the parents to the children, which bred numerous resentments.

After the psychiatrist had interviewed my parents, my husband and I were called in. I was rigid, a non-feeling entity, a robot. My parents stood across from me in the cramped room close to a small side window. They seemed very awkward, as if they didn't want to be there. As nervous as I felt, I began to think this could be my opportunity to stand up to them, where previously that had been too scary. The psychiatrist was at her desk, I was in safer territory. But it was still daunting.

File notes: 2 July '75. Interview with patient's parents – saw them alone for an hour and then with the patient for another hour. The interview proved much more difficult even than anticipated. Father proved more intransigent than Mother, intellectually limited, very defensive in attitude throughout, fixed ideas about everything, and very rambling in his speech. Mother appeared very quick and intelligent and was able to relax as the interview progressed, particularly when she saw that the purpose of the interview was intended to be constructive rather than destructive.

She showed a degree of insight about the lack of communication in the family, and she explained it by commenting that her upbringing was similar, and she thought that it did the children no harm. She admitted that she was a shy person who found it hard to show or express affection.

It appeared that both father and herself had worked hard all their lives to provide for the children. They both considered that this was proof of their concern for the children. It did not seem to occur to them that the children would not see things in exactly the same way. Father repeatedly claimed that the children could always come to him with their problems, but the only examples he cited concerned the eldest son.

When the patient joined the interview and informed them that she had always felt under strain at home because of pressures on her to work, and to study hard without relaxation, her father became defensive. He refused to concede any points and shouted at her several times.

> On the whole, the patient stood up to the interview very well but was inclined to blame her parents for every action of her siblings, seeing things only from their point of view. Possible family interview later on, but doubtful.

Those two sessions were important opportunities for my family and me to explore what had been difficult for all of us in my early life. Everybody had been struggling. Those meetings could have opened the possibility of hearing each other for the first time. But somehow, they didn't appear to change anything. I left the room in floods of tears, thinking things were a hundred times worse than when I had gone in, and that whatever respect my parents might have had for me, it was gone.

My parents seemed angry and aloof at the end of the interview. To me, it seemed as if they were no longer a part of my life and didn't want to be. I had brought shame on my family. I imagine my mother and father especially were mortified, embarrassed and angry.

Reading these reports years later, I was appalled by how my father was described. It's so severe. Lack of intelligence – I found that very hard to read. They just wrote him off, allowing no possibility that maybe he is nice at times, or had any good points.

Two weeks later, I was discharged. The final note in my hospital chart written by my treating psychiatrist read:

> **File notes:** 14 July. Had a number of complaints about the hospital made in a formal fashion, cushioned by assurances that it is a wonderful place and has done wonders for her. Anxious to be off all medication. Maintains that

she has matured and is different now but does not really show any evidence of this. Agreed to attend as an out-patient in Galway.

...

It seems clear that she has a hysterical personality. A detailed history does not reveal that she has ever been of a normal, stable personality, and I advised her husband that there was no question of completely removing her symptoms. My best advice would be that medication should be restricted to small doses of minor tranquillisers and (if this is available) the help of any local psychiatric clinic in your area should be obtained. There is very little I can do to be helpful in a case of this kind. She was initially on fairly high medication with Valium, but we progressively reduced this over a period, and on discharge, she was off all medication. I felt it was important that she should have continuing supportive therapy.'

After my stay at St John of God, to access therapeutic support I travelled 87km to Galway city every Tuesday and Thursday. I attended group therapy in a house across the road from the hospital and felt the better for them. There was no drama. There was nobody who became so visibly upset that I was affected. On the contrary, we often had great fun amongst ourselves and ended up laughing. I felt accepted as a person and on equal terms with everyone. No one viewed me with suspicion. There was a wonderful sense of freedom and respect. The meetings were held in a nice setting, and I could return home afterwards. I was in charge of my own life.

Today, as I reflect on these times, I ask myself what made my life experiences so painful. I felt powerless and had no voice. It wasn't even what they did, it was what they didn't do. They never tried to get to know me as a person. I was talked down to, never asked how I was or what I was feeling. I sense if this had happened, rather than labels being applied that simply suggested there was something wrong with me, I might have found the help I needed.

Interestingly, my first real breakthrough came when I opened up to the priest and fellow patient in St John of God on St Joseph's ward. We just chatted. I felt safe in their company; I felt heard and understood, unlike with the doctors. Sometimes you would find this with the other patients; we were all in the same boat. I cannot remember the priest's name now, but he allowed me to speak as I wanted to without putting me under any pressure to discuss things I didn't want to discuss. He was an alcoholic, and I told Tommy afterwards that some of the nicest people I'd ever met were the alcoholics in that hospital. I felt great after talking to the priest, lighter and relieved after getting it out about the fainting attacks, he was so compassionate.

Today, I can stand up for myself. Being honest and upfront with people is very important to me. Back then, I needed to learn to become happy with myself, change unhelpful thinking patterns that were hurting me and learn to appreciate my gifts, talents and capabilities. I needed to build my confidence and a sense of identity before trying to process what had happened to me in a meaningful way.

Chapter 12

A CRY OF PAIN

Maybe I was 'hysterical', as it said in my files, although I find that a very demeaning term. Or maybe there was a lot of unresolved pain inside me that I expressed physically at times in the absence of having any words to describe it.

I wasn't always in a bad mood. There were also moments of calm, wonder and the satisfaction of a job well done.

After my discharge from 'The Gods', I decided to run a bed and breakfast service for the summer. I recall a day when I was on my hands and knees polishing the dining room floor when I looked up to see the sun streaming through the window. Everything seemed to be transformed, and I was held in awe.

As well as getting the house ready, I made a B&B sign. When we opened for business, I was concerned no one would find us because we lived in a very isolated location. But I needn't have worried. We did exceptionally well. I found the work fulfilling, and the money was welcome. Glowing compliments in the visitors book did wonders for my wellbeing.

When September arrived, we took down the B&B sign. I couldn't wait to return to teaching. But perhaps because the summer work had taken more out of me than I realised, I felt anxious and a little down in myself. My students noticed this. Teenagers don't miss much.

A small group of students began to make what felt like snide remarks when my back was turned. They seemed to be vying with one another about who could come up with the smartest comment. They were sniggering and passing hurtful comments between themselves about the way I was teaching them, as if I was no good as a teacher. The more it went on, the more nervous I became. I desperately wanted them to like me as a teacher and be impressed with my work, but it was all going in the opposite way. I felt ridiculed. I tried to ignore them, but jeering at me became part of the daily classroom routine.

I felt that they were ganging up on me. Now I look back and see they were testing boundaries. They didn't know what was going on in my personal life, but they sensed how vulnerable I was. My inability to make it clear to them that their taunts were unacceptable allowed their behaviour to escalate.

Today, I would handle things differently. With a gentle but firm tone, I would say, 'I'm unhappy with what's going on. Can we talk about this? This behaviour is unacceptable, and my better instincts tell me you're uncomfortable with it, too.'

However, I was a young teacher with poor self-confidence. Instead, I doubled my preparation work, determined to make my classes more interesting. When this strategy didn't make the slightest difference, I couldn't cope. I consulted my GP, who referred me to a psychiatrist at University Hospital, Galway.

I felt that the psychiatrist I met in the outpatient department was cold and abrupt. I described my difficulties in managing my students and how upsetting I had found their comments and insults. His report to my GP read:

Dear Doctor ...

Mrs. O'Toole did not profit much from the psychotherapy received at St John of God Hospital. I believe she is suffering from a 'borderline syndrome' – in that, she was deprived of emotional security in her childhood to such an extent that she is likely to pass through her entire life buying and trading for affection from others. For example, each class she takes has to be a virtuoso performance to earn the admiration and affection of her pupils, after which she will collapse into bed for a day!

In a way, her general behaviour can be looked at as a defence against the risks and dangers of growing up. For Mrs O'Toole to grow up would be to accept that rejection, pain, etc., are part and parcel of life and must be tolerated. She has never believed this and continues to display an insatiable appetite for attention and affection. However, she has improved to the extent that she is able to discuss these things openly.

I believe it may help you in her management if she is seen at this Clinic at intervals of, say, six weeks. We will write regularly and will, of course, see her in any major crisis at short notice.

Yours sincerely,

While it's true that I 'was deprived of emotional security' in my childhood to such an extent that I've spent most of my life in search of affection from other people, his conclusion that I was 'likely to pass through her entire life buying and trading for affection from others' feels insulting. It dismissed any potential in me to grow and change.

For over 40 years, I have taught in schools, and I currently teach the piano privately and prepare students for the Royal Irish Academy of Music exams. I have not put my heart and soul into teaching, producing musicals and directing choirs to impress people. I have worked hard, particularly with young people, out of my passionate love for music and a genuine desire to ensure that each student enjoys the process and is successful in their efforts.

Yes, I've had my issues. In spite of my best efforts, they have, at times, overwhelmed me, and I've needed to withdraw or allow myself to be cared for by others. But most of the time, I've made a conscious choice to live my life as courageously as I could. And to do so with integrity.

To write off my entire personality as a defence against 'the risks and dangers of growing up' is simplistic and untrue. I know full well that rejection and pain are part of life. I learned that lesson early on and have spent my life since coming to terms with it.

I had better control of the class when I returned to school. I was doing very well until a critical incident rocked the entire community. One of my students was killed when his bicycle was hit by a car. I knew that student and his family very well. I found his death very upsetting and couldn't stop thinking about him and his family. When my grief persisted and took away my sleep, I made an appointment to return to the Department of Psychiatry in Galway. This time I met with a younger man, who wrote back to my GP:

15 December, '75

Ms O'Toole has been coping with her job for three or four weeks following her last visit here. Since then, she has become depressed, tense and anxious and feels unable to continue working. This she tells me is due to the fact that one of her pupils was killed in a road accident and this upset her very much … she has been very depressed and insomniac for several nights. She expresses ideas of futility. In view of this, I have given her a prescription for Tryptizol 25mg twice daily, 50mg at night. I think that she ought to continue on Tryptizol for about a month. By that time, I would hope her depression would have lifted and that she will again be able to cope.

Kind regards.

Yours sincerely …

I returned to work in the hope that the drugs would eventually work. My depression didn't lift, but I stopped taking medication when I discovered I was pregnant. I was delighted, but a month later, I experienced a shock that completely unnerved me.

On a cold day in January 1976, I was at home when I heard a commotion in the hall. Next thing, I saw Tommy coming through the front door with many of our neighbours behind him. Usually, he always came in the side door. I braced myself. He looked troubled. Everyone else had their heads down. I was so conscious of the little baby – I was four months pregnant. I thought, *I'm not going to let anything affect this baby, I don't care what it is.*

I didn't know what was coming.

Tommy approached me – he was very gentle, but the shock in his face scared me, because I'd never seen anything like it in Tommy before – and said, 'Breda, your father has been killed in a tragic accident. Last night, a bad storm uprooted a tree on your uncle's farm. The fallen tree needed to be cleared. Your dad offered to help. After driving your mother to the hospital, where she was booked in for major surgery, he went directly to assist your uncle. High up in the tree about to cut down another branch, he fell, hit the main road, and was killed instantly.'

A physical shock ran straight down my body from my head to my toes. Commotion followed. We drove to Limerick immediately and headed straight for the funeral parlour. My dad laid out in a coffin felt unreal. I stumbled back to where Tommy was standing. He took me in his arms. I couldn't stop crying. There were tensions in the family home which made everything worse. Tommy knew I was uncomfortable, and we got away as fast as we could afterwards.

The good thing about it was my father died saving people's lives. It was tragic for us, but what a beautiful way to die.

The extraordinary thing about my father, that I cannot say about my mother, was I always had a soft spot for my dad. No matter what he did, I still had a soft spot for him. Okay, there were times when I came back, and it was as if I didn't exist in that house. But there was still something. Maybe it all went back to that day when he taught us 'Silent Night', and I saw another side of him. Or making Christmas decorations when we were children – just paper streamers, as that's all anyone could afford – but I'd see a happy man, the gloom and doom was going and something bright and beautiful came into our house. In those kinds of moments, I saw a side of him that endeared me to him. Or him to me.

In Limerick when I was growing up, he'd occasionally say he was going to the creamery (a good few miles away) for milk, and he'd ask would I like to come. I'd be in my element. Those were lovely times. He wasn't drunk. He was more at home with himself. All those moments build up in you. I was fond of him. Terrified of him, of that other man. But also fond of him. That's why his death came as such a blow to me.

I was glad to be away from the aggro, but at the end of the day, your dad is your dad. It was so unexpected, because he wasn't sick.

Four weeks later, I had a miscarriage. Tommy rushed me to the maternity hospital in Galway. The consultant gynaecologist, the same man who had looked after me with Dermot, told me the baby had died when I heard about my father's death. 'It was because you were so determined to hang on that you only miscarried now.'

I lay motionless in the bed in a dreadful state. I longed for someone to talk to, but nobody was around. I could see how busy the nurses were, so I didn't want to bother them with requests to talk. Finally, I asked a nurse if she could send word to the psychiatric unit to let them know I had been admitted following the death of my child, hoping that someone might come to talk to me in the ward where I was.

Not long after, a male psychiatrist in a white coat arrived at my bedside. He stood, a silent, upright figure, looking down at my file. He appeared cold and clinical. He looked up and quizzed me about previous admissions to psychiatric hospitals. I wondered, *Why is he talking down to me? Does he not know I've just had a miscarriage?* I was shocked when he announced abruptly that he was transferring me to the psychiatric unit.

The last place I wanted to go was the psychiatric unit, but I was afraid to say anything in case that would go against me. I regret now that I didn't stand my ground. Instead, I handed control of my life over to the psychiatrist. Today, I wouldn't allow anyone to do that.

A few days later, I was discharged and soon returned to teaching. Given the distress we'd both experienced in attempting to have a child, Tommy and I began to think about adoption. We contacted the adoption agency and went through a very thorough vetting process. I was very open with the social worker and told her I'd suffered from depression. 'That's not a problem,' she said, 'but I will need a letter of recommendation from the psychiatrist who treated you to finalise the papers.'

I made an appointment to see him, confident that he would agree. He refused. I explained that we had been successful in all the interviews and home visits, the Social Services were in favour, and we just needed a letter from him to finalise proceedings. He replied, 'You will have to remain of stable temperament for nine months first.'

Medical Report: 24 May, '76.

Dear Doctor …

Mrs. O'Toole is not very pleased with me, particularly for opposing adoption. I rather discouraged her when I saw her recently from remaining in psychiatric care. I told her that her cyclical tension symptoms were very likely related to menstruation and that she ought to seek further opinion on this. She is a rather unhappy, neurotic person, and I doubt if continued psychiatric attendance will benefit her to any great extent. I assured her that I would be willing to support a further application to adopt a child provided that she had been of stable temperament for at least nine months previously. She may or may not return for review.

 Yours sincerely,

There are tears in my eyes over how I was treated that day. His manner towards me was appalling. What stood out most for me was his power. I always felt belittled and insignificant in his company at every appointment I attended, but this was worse. I wasn't allowed to question his authority, not for a second.

While I can appreciate and acknowledge that I had lived through a traumatic 18 months and that asking me to wait nine months was reasonable and good medical practice, there was something about the way he told me that left me feeling downgraded and trampled upon. His manner communicated that I had no say in the matter whatsoever.

I tried to put my opinion across, but he became even more belligerent. What a pity the matter wasn't discussed between us on equal terms in a civil and acceptable manner, and both of us agreed on the final decision to wait.

I found some of the psychiatrists under whose care I spent time to be men enclosed within their own power, a world unto themselves. Godlike, in their own esteem. In my dealings with some of them, I was greeted with an attitude of, *I'm the one who knows everything here, you listen to me and do what I tell you.*

No appointment lasted more than ten minutes, I find it hard to see how you would learn much from a person who has come to you looking for help in that short time.

I was in a dark place when I left that office that day. Over the past 18 months, our first baby had died, my father was killed in a tragic accident, and a month later I had a miscarriage. Somehow, I managed to keep going. A month later, we opened for B&B.

In September 1976, the start of the new school year, I returned to teaching. By then, I was a tormented soul. I was in a vulnerable place and couldn't think clearly about anything. I had very little, if any, self-awareness. Derogatory thoughts circled around and around in my head. I didn't know how to deal with them. I was in a mental prison that I couldn't escape from.

Whatever the beatings I endured as a child, I was the one now beating myself up. What a difference now. Today, I take increasing responsibility for my moods and behaviours. I make determined efforts not to let unhelpful thoughts or low mood levels get the upper hand.

I kept going until the end of that year, but by January 1977, I'd reached a new low point. After a particularly rough day in school, I sat in my car as intense emotions of fear, helplessness, and despair swept through my body. I started to think about suicide. I couldn't make sense of what was happening and felt I'd lost control of my life. Suicide felt like the only way to take back control, to stop the pain finally.

Unsure of what to do, I turned the ignition key and drove towards town. I pulled up at the priest's house. The side door was open. Mustering all the courage I had, I overheard voices from an inner room. Men were talking about golf. The priest noticed me and immediately invited me in. But I was embarrassed and replied, 'Father, it's okay; I'll come back again.' I didn't want to intrude. I thanked him and left.

Back in the car, I could barely hold it together. I knew I couldn't return home in that state. I drove to the nearest off-licence. I ordered a bottle each of brandy, whiskey and Irish Mist liqueur. I made my way back to the car and drove home. Luckily, there was no one there. I headed straight for the bedroom.

I opened the bottle of liqueur and gulped down enough to put me to sleep. I placed the three bottles in the wardrobe and got into bed. Every time I woke, I went to the wardrobe and drank a few more mouthfuls until all three were gone. I returned to bed, convinced I would never wake up again.

At some point, I did wake up. I was still alive. Struggling out of bed, I groped along the bedroom wall and went to the kitchen. I opened the kitchen cabinet to my right and pulled out a container of Anadin painkiller tablets. I counted 40 into my hand, swallowed the whole lot with a glass of milk and returned to my bed. This time, there was no coming back.

But at some point, my eyes flickered open. When I realised I was still alive, I sat up in the bed. The enormity of what I had done hit me. Shock sensations ran through my body as I realised, I didn't want to die. I was terrified. What had I done?

Susan, my sister, was here on holiday. Too scared and

ashamed to call Tommy, I shouted her name several times. I told her about the three bottles of alcohol and 40 Anadin I had taken. She called Tommy, who rushed into the room, worry written all over his face. He bent down, cupped his hands around my face and said, 'Breda, I love you.' Those three words gave me back the will to live.

The GP was called and reassured Tommy that there was every chance I could recover. But he added, 'It's too late to pump her out. Try to get her to vomit by putting her fingers down her throat or drinking salted water.' I cooperated but couldn't vomit. Tommy phoned the doctor again, who said, 'She'll be okay, but she will have violent bodily reactions during the night. It's more than likely convulsions, too. Just stay with her. With your support, she can come through it.'

Tommy and I lived through a terrifying night. The involuntary, violent spasms contorted my body into all sorts of unusual shapes and angles. At times, my body bounced up and down into the air. But that night, I found an inner strength that enabled me to remain calm until everything quietened again. Tommy was at my side. That was all I needed. As a new dawn appeared outside the window, I fell asleep.

The next day, I was readmitted to St John of God Hospital. Tommy and I were hardly inside the door when the receptionist said, 'Because you're an alcoholic, you must go to the alcoholic unit.' I was shocked. I tried to explain that even though I had taken so much alcohol the previous day, I had never done so ever before in my life. She didn't believe me. Tommy intervened and backed me up. His words were brushed aside.

A nurse escorted me to the alcohol unit and locked me in

their isolation room. A small room with bare white walls. I sat on the edge of the chair in the middle of the floor. I was terrified, feeling completely powerless. My body was cold and shaking. After a long time, a psychiatrist entered the room, interviewed me, and locked the door when she left. I was treated for 'modified withdrawal' from alcohol for three days with Heminevrin, a sedative used to treat symptoms of acute alcohol withdrawal.

> **File notes:** 13 Jan, '77. Admitted on a voluntary basis, accompanied by her husband. The patient was tired, pale and cold on admission and very tense and anxious. Seen and examined by Doctor .... During this time, she displayed dramatic, attention-seeking and hysterical behaviour, for example, shaking and complaining of fainting. Slept all night.

Three days later, a nurse took me to the day room. She let me in and then locked the door. I glanced around and saw groups of patients sitting in a smoky atmosphere, doing nothing. I spotted an empty chair, sat down and kept my distance.

The only thing I could do was observe. I could hardly see through the heavy haze in the room. By evening, my surroundings had become intolerable. Men were vomiting on the floor. There was no one to clean up. Other patients ranted and raved. Noise levels became deafening as the day progressed. For the first time, I witnessed uproar and chaotic behaviour. I wanted to run, but there was no escape.

When a nurse eventually returned me to my room, I dared

not say a word. I knew better than to complain. If I said anything, I always had the risk of being heavily medicated.

The next day, 17 January 1977, I was transferred to St Joseph's ward on the condition that I would attend the Alcohol Withdrawal Programme. From an intellectual point of view, I appreciated the lectures. One evening, I saw a young girl with shoulder-length black hair playing the piano with bandages on her lower arms. Another patient said she had slit her wrists. For some reason, I found this very upsetting.

That night, I couldn't sleep. At 4 a.m., I approached the nurses' station. The woman behind the desk glanced up sternly and said, 'What do you want?' I replied, 'I can't sleep.' She seemed annoyed with me. 'You're not the only one in the world who can't sleep,' she said. I went back to bed. The next day, I pretended to be well to get out of the place. Three days later, I asked to be discharged.

> **File notes:** 20 January '77. The patient has asked for discharge this weekend following a conversation with her husband on the phone. Feels she is ready to go and wishes to see Doctor … regarding the same. Slept very well without medication.

Before leaving the hospital, Tommy and I were interviewed by the medical director. He addressed me and said, 'You do not have an alcohol problem. You drank for escape reasons only. However, I would like to caution you that if you continue down that road, you will indeed become an alcoholic.' At no time did anyone ask me what had led to me making a suicide attempt.

Discharge summary: 31 Jan, '77

Dear Doctor ...

Thank you for referring Mrs. O'Toole, who was admitted here on 13 January 1977. Her presenting complaint was anxiety and inability to cope with frequent hysterical manifestations. She has also been abusing alcohol and sedatives of late. You will remember that she had been treated for a similar problem in 1975. She seems to have coped reasonably well since then, her recent illness being precipitated by the death of her father, followed by a miscarriage a month later.

She responded well to psychotherapy and mild tranquillisers. As she was anxious to get off all medication, we gradually reduced the dose, and she was discharged on no medication on 22 January 1977. We have advised that she continue seeing Doctor ... and would attend the day centre attached to his unit one day a week. I feel this would give her the support and help she needs to reduce the frequency of her hysterical outbursts. I am afraid the prognosis must remain guarded in this case.

Yours sincerely,

After I was discharged from St John of God Hospital, I attended the Psychiatric Unit in Galway once a week as an outpatient. My health continued to deteriorate.

File notes: Psychiatric Unit, UHG 9 March, '77

Dear Doctor …

This lady is suffering from an anxiety state with hysterical reactions. She was seen at our Day Care Centre here for a few days. However, [her psychiatrist] thinks that this lady has a chronic personality problem and that recurrence is quite likely, and he would discourage long-term psychiatric care, so he has discharged her from our care.

One afternoon, after I had done the food shopping, I was overwhelmed by horrible physical feelings. My body had gone stiff and was shutting down. By now frantic over what was happening to me, I was forced to stop. I knew I couldn't keep driving and that if I tried to reach home, just a stone's throw away, I would be in danger of crashing the car. I pulled the car off the road and turned off the ignition. Sitting there, feeling utterly without hope, I couldn't take any more. My body was making weird shapes I had no control over, and I was shaking viciously.

I had spent five years attending psychiatric hospitals, where apart from St Vincent's psychiatric unit, the regime was harsh and cruel. Nothing had worked. I felt no one understood what I was going through, not even Tommy. The intense mental and emotional pain I felt inwardly, coupled with my body not functioning, was more than I could cope with. Terrified, I told myself, *There's no suffering in heaven. I have to reach God.*

I drove to the beach and parked the car. Resolutely, I walked to the edge of the sea and kept walking. As the waters swirled around me, I closed my eyes. The more I moved forward, the more I was pleasantly surprised by the deep peace surrounding me. I kept moving forward.

I got a fright when my shoulders were grabbed roughly from behind. I spluttered, lost my balance, and gasped for air. I had no idea who was pulling me back in such a rough, heavy-handed way. I didn't realise it was Tommy until I heard his voice. To this day, he doesn't remember how he happened to be there. I think stress has caused gaps in his memory too. I wonder now if he was on high alert about where I was.

With a firm hold on my hand, we struggled, step by step, as the swirling incoming tide made it hard to reach the shore. I was furious at Tommy for rescuing me. A surge of overpowering emotions that I had never felt before consumed me. Deep-seated anger, hatred, dark despair, confusion, fear. I didn't recognise the person I had become.

Unable to speak, I recall sitting in the passenger seat. Tommy glanced over at me. Neither of us spoke. He drove up the road. Inside the house, I went to the bedroom, took off my wet clothes, returned to the sitting room, and curled up on the couch, numb. After a long time, I fell asleep.

Thankfully, Tommy didn't tell the doctor but allowed me to recover in my own time. In the days after, we never discussed what had happened. I was too ashamed. What did Tommy think of me, the lowest of the low? If anything, I wanted to be left alone.

I was struggling, trying to survive from minute to minute. As I drove into town a few weeks later, I was overwhelmed, once again, by indescribable physical sensations. I understand now that I was having a panic attack. In a fit of desperation, I drove the car recklessly over the edge of an embankment near my aunt-in-law's house. I vaguely remember being pulled out of the car by some men who brought me to her home. Neighbours gathered, and I was put lying flat on the couch. When anyone asked me what had happened, I said, 'The car went out of control.' I couldn't be honest. The risk of returning to a psychiatric hospital was too distressing. The doctor arrived, checked me out, and was satisfied that I was okay. He left a prescription for Valium tranquillisers. Tommy drove me home later that evening.

Victor Frankl, a renowned psychiatrist held prisoner in Auschwitz and other concentration camps, states: 'A man's concern, even his despair, over the worthwhileness of life is an *existential distress* but by no means a *mental disease.*'* I couldn't agree more. That is my lived experience.

---

* Frankl, Viktor E., *Man's Search For Meaning: An Introduction to Logotherapy.* Preface by Gordon W. Allport. Simon & Schuster, New York.

Chapter 13

FINDING HOPE

I wish I could describe the dark, oppressive mood I was in that early afternoon in March 1977, just before Tommy entered the kitchen. It was days after my third suicide attempt. I was standing over the range, lost in time, with no idea how to continue with life in any shape or form. I heard his voice behind me saying, 'Breda, would you like to go on a holiday?' Astonished, I turned sideways and replied, 'Do you mean it? Where?' He nodded and said, 'Yes, but where we're going is a surprise.' I didn't care. I wanted to get out of Ireland.

I can still see us both sitting halfway back on the plane in my mind's eye. I hadn't a clue where we were going. When we were at the airport, I was too highly unwell to take notice of what was going on in my surroundings. I think Tommy checked in the bags while I just stood there motionless beside him. I reached down to take a book out of my bag, but froze when a priest stood at the front of the plane and invited everyone to join him in saying the rosary.

I did not want to go on a pilgrimage. My only thought was, *Let me off this plane.* My eyes caught sight of the exit door, but obviously, I couldn't jump out. I was enclosed in a space I didn't want to be in. Faith or anything to do with religion meant nothing to me at that time. My life up to that point had sabotaged any hope of finding a spirituality to sustain me during dark times.

We were on our way to Lourdes, a small village in the foothills of the Pyrenees Mountains in France. On 11 February 1858,

Bernadette Soubirous, a 14-year-old peasant girl, experienced the first of 18 apparitions. She had gone to Massabielle to collect firewood. A rush of wind caught her attention, and when she looked over towards a nearby cave, she noticed a white figure, 'a beautiful lady' who later described herself as 'The Immaculate Conception'.

Miracles – officially declared by the International Medical Committee of Lourdes (CMIL) – have occurred there ever since. People have been cured of cancer, lung disease, skin problems, paralysis, physical disabilities, etc. Millions flock to the international Marian shrine every year.

After we arrived at Tarbes-Lourdes-Pyrenees Airport, we boarded a coach to Lourdes, 11km away. We were staying in Hôtel Jeanne d'Arc, situated in the heart of the village, a short distance from the prominent sanctuaries. We settled in, and after breakfast the following morning, we met up with the rest of the group, staying in nearby hotels. The priest read out the daily itinerary.

Being unable to stand and listen while pretending I was well was a constant strain. One day, as we were heading back to the hotel, a group came down the street reciting the rosary. I was annoyed at the repetitious sound of the prayers. When they came closer, I saw the devoted look on their faces. I didn't share their belief, but I sensed their faith as if I could feel it in the air around me.

I looked forward to the torchlight processions at night. No matter how terrible I felt, the atmosphere, the singing, everything about the processions lifted me. I recall the night that loud cracks of thunder and incredible flashes of lightning, followed by a deluge of rain that soaked the streets, didn't stop us. We grabbed umbrellas, and off we went.

As we walked along the route carrying lighted candles, it was amazing to see different countries represented, with pilgrims carrying eye-catching banners shoulder high. The rosary was recited in various languages, and in between each decade, everyone joined in singing the Lourdes Hymn. I loved the sense of unity in our shared humanity.

There were countless sick people, many in wheelchairs. I was unwell, but at least I was able to move around. We attended Mass in the underground Basilica of Saint Pius X. I loved being there. The atmosphere, music, and choirs were a lovely reprieve from my ill health.

One night, as we returned to the hotel after a singsong, we decided to go to the grotto. As we entered, I was touched by the deep peace.

At the shrine, Tommy said, 'I want to go and light some candles.' I wasn't interested and replied, 'You go; I'll wait here.' I stood motionless, not knowing what to do. I was too sick to go anywhere. I began to think about Our Lady and what the grotto was about. I had no relationship with her. I felt an emptiness inside.

I turned my face, looked up at the statue and said, 'Okay. If you're in it, then let me get pregnant.' After the death of our first and second baby, I had been trying for over two years without success. When Tommy came back, we walked around the grotto, slowly and in silence. I loved the peace – the stillness.

The following day, we went with the group to see St Bernadette's birthplace: the Moulin de Boly, in the centre of Lourdes. Bernadette was born in this watermill on 7 January 1844.

On day four, we visited the baths, which date back to the 18th century. Their source is the original spring, which Bernadette discovered at the Massabielle grotto during the ninth apparition on 25 February 1858. The waters are believed to be a source of great healing. Total immersion, with the help of attendees, lasts for a couple of minutes. Tommy and I braved the freezing waters.

The next day I felt unwell, but still enjoyed the trip up to Pic du Jer, a French Pyrenean summit on a cable railway system that overlooks the town of Lourdes from 950 metres (3,120 feet).

Early the following day, we returned to Ireland. After we landed in Dublin, I convinced Tommy to buy me a knitting machine. I needed something to do. I had decided to retire from teaching on health grounds. I was receiving sick leave payment from the Department of Education. I was entitled to it as a fully qualified teacher, but I felt guilt-ridden at taking money while I was unable to work for months (some of this was imbued by the Catholic teachings I had grown up with). That was soul-destroying, really demoralising.

For the next few weeks, the knitting machine took up most of my time. Figuring out how to use it and working hard to make children's sweaters and a V-necked jumper for Tommy, gave me something to focus on.

Halfway through making Tommy's sweater, another idea formed in my mind. I considered staging a concert as a fund-raiser and involving the local schoolchildren. I approached the teachers in both national schools. They were delighted, as were the parents. In hindsight, even though I appeared confident, my self-esteem was low. I doubted my ability. I worried that no one would show up for rehearsals. I was fearful the children didn't like me and became obsessed with what others thought of me. I pushed myself to extremes to have everything right so that I would be admired. Everything had to be perfect.

I held the rehearsals in the community hall at weekends. I made the costumes and props. The highlight of the show was the song 'Puff the Magic Dragon'. A schoolteacher offered to make the dragon. The night was a tremendous success, and the proceeds went to a local charity. Afterwards, I stood alone on the stage behind the curtain, unsure that my efforts had been appreciated. But I learned an important lesson. Whenever I'm at a performance, I try to go up afterwards to congratulate those involved and express my gratitude.

That summer before opening for B&B, I applied for membership in the Bord Fáilte Farmhouse Association. A lady came to inspect our house and was pleased with what she saw. I was surprised to hear we had to provide our guests with an evening meal and breakfast. I asked five girls in the locality to work on shifts. I appreciated what it was like to work hard without pay, and I was determined that these girls would be well rewarded.

Nothing gave me more pleasure than cordon bleu cuisine, which I learned from magazines. To this day, I take great pleasure in creating delicious meals. From my experience of the food in one psychiatric institution, I swore I'd never serve meals like that to anyone.

For our guests, we specialised in fresh seafood, lobster and shellfish from local fishermen. We also had a wine licence, and our reputation grew as a great place to stay. I was amazed when I read a glowing tribute in France's leading newspaper, *Le Monde*, and also in a Dutch magazine.

In late June, I discovered I was two months pregnant. I had been afraid to think I might be. When I attended the gynaecologist, he assured me that the baby was due on 2 January 1978 and because of my history, he wouldn't let me go past that date.

One day that summer, the local priest popped in for a visit during the tourist season. He chatted away for a while, then said, 'Breda, will you do the music in the church for me?' 'Father, I'm sorry. I can't.' The priest didn't know I had been through 29 electric shock treatments and could no longer play. Because of the repeated ECTs, I lost my ability to play the piano. I had realised this at the time, sitting down at the piano one day – playing would have been calming for me, and something I did daily – everything was blank, there was nothing there, I had no recall whatsoever. Until the day I go to the grave, I will remain horror-struck over this significant loss in my life.

I had reached university standard, but everything I had learned was lost.

There's a grief deep inside me that won't go away – years of the best of professional instrumental training and learning gone down the drain. In addition, for decades, I endured constant pain in both temples where the electrodes were placed.

As the priest left that day, he turned and said, 'Breda, I'm buying you an organ. I mean it!' As the day wore on, I felt terrible. I didn't want to let him down. I found a hymn book, sat at the piano, and began teaching myself a few simple hymns. Early beginnings led me to form an adult and children's choir and learn challenging accompaniments to accompany a local tenor for weddings and funerals.

In 2005 I decided to teach the piano privately at home and

I've been doing so ever since. Each year, my students have consistently been awarded Honours and Distinctions in the Royal Irish Academy of Music grade examinations.

Mid-June 2024, I started learning the piano again, determined to regain my ability to play and reclaim the gift that music had always been for me. Day after day, I would practise. I wanted to perform Grade 8 pieces. I eventually achieved my goal.

When my Fiona and Karen, our eldest daughters, were in secondary school, they needed help with their maths. When I was going through the school system, maths was my lifeline. The one thing I had to hold onto was I was absolutely brilliant at maths. Top of the class, and I loved it. That was one thing in my life where people could look up to me. But when the girls asked me for help with their homework, I was just gutted. I looked at the page, there was nothing that I could recall. As a mother, that was even more painful than losing the music. This was my children. I've never gotten that back.

I learned Italian for three years in the convent. When I went to college I did it for a year. I can't recall a word of Italian. It's gone. It can be hard to come to terms with these losses connected to a treatment that I found entirely unhelpful.

On 2 January 1978, our eldest daughter Fiona was born. Finally, a longed-for child. But I hadn't a clue about babies. Breastfeeding was discouraged and regarded as a taboo subject. There were few supports in place for first-time mothers. My daughter had a click in her hips, and I was told that each time I changed her, I would have to put on three Terry cloth nappies, but no explanation was given. The *amount* of extra washing!

When I got home, I stood in the front room of our home in Connemara, frozen. I had never felt as helpless in my life. I was feeling far from well. I didn't know how to sterilise or make up bottles. I was unsure how to put on the three nappies at a time correctly. I had never bathed a baby. In the hospital, there had been no instruction. Just at that moment, the doorbell rang. I rushed out to open the front door. My friend Bernie was standing there. I was never so delighted to see anyone in my life. She came in, took over and showed me the basics; I didn't even know how to make a bottle. My God, did she know what to do; she saved the day for me. She was kind and loving and took the time to explain.

My only regret is that I didn't know more about colic and how that affects a baby. I knew nothing about it. I thought I was a bad mother, because I couldn't stop my child crying. I wandered the house for three months, thinking I was a lousy mother. There were days when the baby kept crying for hours, and I was home all day on my own with her. I thought that was my fault. I found that soul-destroying. Today, there's medication available for colic, but back then, the only thing on the market was gripe water. In my daughter's case, that rarely made a difference. She would just cry and cry. There might be two or three hours' break in the evening, and then it would start up again. I hadn't been able to breastfeed, so even unconsciously, I felt I had failed at that. I wasn't aware that the lack of sleep involved in having a newborn would be having a further detrimental effect on my mental health.

Our second eldest daughter, Karen, was born 11 months later the same year, on 5 December 1978. By then, breastfeeding was encouraged in the hospital as long as we did it in the room down the corridor. I couldn't wait to get home. After all, I had learned to mind our first daughter; I felt pretty confident. Sometime later, I stood in the hall at home for a moment and savoured the feeling of how much I was enjoying looking after them both.

But motherhood didn't come easy to me. When our first baby, Dermot, died, I felt ashamed and guilty because of what had happened. Most of all, I felt a deep void, a heartache that I hadn't had a chance to bond with him. My unresolved grief kept coming back to bite me. Had I gotten the dates wrong? Was I responsible for his death? My remorse gnawed away inside me. I was always good at providing for their material needs, but I found the emotional side of parenting more challenging.

To my surprise, I thoroughly enjoyed the experience of raising my babies. Tommy very occasionally liked to go for a pint with the lads, but I wasn't into drinking. I didn't like the pub scene, especially because of associations with my father. Even on my wedding day, when I saw all the men gathered around the bar, I cringed.

It was mostly getting through each day here. When we got married, and our kids were young, there wasn't as much demand for building houses as there would be nowadays. If there was a wet day, they couldn't work, and there are a lot of wet days in Connemara where we live. We had very little money to begin with, but even less when Tommy's work was rained off. Often people would be slow to pay him for the work he had done. I remember one Christmas Eve going around with him to various houses, because we hadn't a penny, and the only hope we had was that he would collect the money he was owed from the people he had been working for. When our first two daughters were young, money was very tight. Tommy was asked one day to do a carpentry job in a supply store in town. He would have grabbed work from anywhere, we were so desperate. He did that job, and never left, giving up building houses to work in the shop. I only found out years later he was very unhappy. Not because of where he was working, but it wasn't him. He wanted to be outside, building houses in the fresh air, but he sacrificed that for his family, so there would be a steady income every week. This just shows his character. He's amazing.

After I got up in the mornings it was mostly about getting through each day at home. I didn't have any social life as it wasn't my scene. I felt awkward in the company of others, always on edge.

People used to call Fiona and Karen twins, because they were born so close together. By the time Karen arrived, I felt an expert on babies. I really enjoyed looking after the two kids at that stage. I felt I had a natural spontaneity with them. I loved taking pictures of them in the front room, that kind of thing.

But as the girls grew older, mothering became harder for me. Nothing had prepared me for the 'terrible twos'. My childhood had been impoverished, leaving me ill-equipped to know what to do. I was convinced I was just no good at child-rearing.

As much as I could, I tried to put on a brave face and appear 'normal', but behind the mask, my children didn't have the mother they deserved. There were times when I wished I could explain my ill health to them, but I hadn't the words to describe it in a way they would understand. I was deeply ashamed of the damage I was doing to their young minds.

When they started school, I had at least some time to myself. But between collecting them from school and Tommy arriving home from work, I wasn't confident about how to deal with them. There were many days when I locked the kitchen door as the only way I had to cope with being so unwell and so that I could get things done like cooking the dinner. I couldn't bear my children to see me in the terrible state I was in. More often than not I was cooking the meals through a haze of tears. I always ensured they were safe in the front room, watching TV, playing in their bedrooms or the long hall.

One day, in the throes of my inadequacy, while driving past the church, I noticed another young mother on her way to the shop. I knew her. I was distraught with worry and needed to talk to someone. I was so conscious of having two young girls at home who needed me, and I was so worried about the effect my being so sick was having on them. At that point I wasn't able to reach out and hug them to express my love for them. I pulled up alongside her, wound down the window, and after we chatted for a couple of minutes, she said, 'Breda, are you okay? You look worried.'

I admitted, 'Yes, I am worried. I don't love my children.' She paused for a moment. Then, in a kind, gentle, affirming way, she said, 'But of course you love your children. You wouldn't be telling me you don't if you didn't deeply care.' What she said had a profound impact on me that day; it was very reassuring.

Some months later, I opened up to our local priest, a former psychiatric nurse, and told him how concerned I was that my poor health was damaging my two children. He looked at me with a broad smile and said, 'Breda, you are not causing the damage you think you are.' He continued, 'Regardless of your health, they live in a loving environment. Even when you're not up to being there for them in the way you long to be able to do, those girls are surrounded by the love they're getting from Tommy, from their grandparents who live next door, and they're always back and over to them, from neighbours up and down the road, their friends in and out of school. I've seen it. You do not need to worry. Just keep doing the best you can.'

Soon afterwards, I heard of a parenting course to start in Galway, the first of its kind, run by a Jesuit priest, Father Paul. I signed up and travelled weekly to Galway. I have good memories of being a part of that group, it felt like being with people who spoke the same language; everyone was experiencing difficulties with parenting, there was no judgement. The meetings were held in a bright, uplifting room. The atmosphere was loving and friendly. A few dads were also present. Among the skills we were taught, the two I remember most are active listening and the importance of 'I' messages. It was as if we were all there for one another. I thrived as never before. I got to know Paul well and opened up a bit to him. He stayed in contact with me, and that friendship developed.

I had thought that children had to do what their parents told them. If they objected in any way, I felt depleted as a mother and ended up giving out to myself that I didn't have what it takes to be a good mother.

But the course showed me how to look at things differently. I learned that squabbles are a natural daily occurrence in most homes. I felt reassured that I wasn't alone. What was happening to me as a parent was happening to others too. It wasn't the end of the world.

I discovered a new skill that would enable me to listen to my children in a more heartfelt way, to really listen and not be trying to do other things at the same time. It's called active listening. For example, my response to a child's concerns and even those of an adult can be, 'I can see you're upset. Would you like to talk about this?' If the child or person in my company says ' No' then I need to honour and respect that reply. They may not be ready to talk about it.

We did a lot of role play. We divided up into groups of two, each participant facing the other. One adult would act boisterous, give out, or maybe share that he/she had been bullied that day in school, for example. The other's job was to sit and listen and feed back what he/she was saying so that the child felt seen, heard and understood. Where required, as in the case of bullying, to let the child know that he/she wouldn't stand for that and would have a chat with the teacher. That way the child would feel safe and protected.

Mostly, I learned to mother by watching how Tommy loved our children. Not that I was able to copy him right away. I envied his ability to sit in the armchair and enjoy their company while I stayed busy, which was how I survived.

Chapter 14

OVERCOMING VALIUM ADDICTION

In late 1979, Pope John Paul II visited Ireland. Along with thousands of others, Tommy and I went to see him speak in Ballybrit Racecourse, Galway. We walked for miles, then sat for hours, squatting on the ground waiting for him to appear. I was so sick, but the one thing you don't want is for anyone to see how bad you are, for fear you will be written off as insane. It was all about burying what you were actually going through, putting all your energy into making sure nobody notices, because you want to appear normal. The event gave me a temporary lift, but as the year ended, and a new decade began, I was still feeling awful and relying heavily on Valium.

Someone wise wrote: 'As long as you keep secrets and suppress the information, you are fundamentally at war with yourself.'* Talking about my ten-year furtive addiction to Valium tranquillisers is my way of declaring that war is over.

I used to swallow Valium pills like sweets. Some days, I managed by taking Valium 5mg, but more often than not, I needed Valium 10mg. In the 1970s and 1980s, there was no problem getting repeat prescriptions. After buying the pills from the chemist, I used to bring them home and hide them around the house. Many times, I tried to give them up but couldn't.

---

* Van Der Kolk, Bessel. *The Body Keeps the Score*. Penguin Random House UK, 2014, p.278.

One day in the middle of summer 1979, I begged God, 'Please, let me see the day when I throw them in the fire.'

I needed the Valium to keep going. Whenever I got tensed up, when things got too much, when I felt my head was about to crack from high levels of chronic anxiety and I didn't know where to turn, that's when Valium kept me going. I knew I needed a certain amount each day to keep me at equilibrium if I was to have any hope at all. There was nobody near me I could talk to, nobody who understood what I was living through. Valium was my lifesaver.

Earlier that year, Tommy had built an extension to our home. We had five bedrooms available for guests. I worked hard daily, caring for my family and the business. When I felt under pressure, I grabbed Valium. Unexpectedly, to my horror, I woke so unwell one morning in late August that I couldn't move. No matter how hard I tried, I could not get out of bed.

To my shame, I was in such a wrong way that Tommy had to take off work to cook breakfasts for the guests. I felt guilty. I was unable to function, but instead of being compassionate towards myself, in my head, I kept giving out about how useless I was. I drifted in and out of sleep.

Every time I woke, I felt worse than before. I slipped my hand underneath the pillow to take more Valium. By evening, I could hardly function. I felt dreadful. The Valium hadn't worked. I dragged myself out of bed and made it to the front room. In desperation, I flung the last bottle of Valium into the fire. I don't remember how I got through the next couple of days, but I woke up one morning feeling much better, and my health steadily improved after that.

The Clifden Pony Show had taken place, the tourist season was over, and we could return to our bedrooms. Then, the unexpected happened. Two weeks to the day after throwing the Valium in the fire, I woke suspended in the air.

I yelled out, 'I've lost my mind. Look, I'm up here.' Tommy replied, 'What are you talking about? You're right beside me.' Petrified, I said, 'No, I'm not. I'm up here.' He jumped up, leaned over me, looked me straight in the eye, and in the most gentle, tender voice I've ever heard, he said, 'Breda, it must be withdrawal symptoms. It has to be.'

There was a telling silence before he spoke again: 'Breda, I'll tell you this. Over the years, you have proved time and time again that you can do anything you want. You can get through this, too.'

He got dressed and phoned the doctor to find out the withdrawal symptoms associated with Valium. The doctor didn't know.

The following morning, I happened to be in the kitchen when I heard an interview on the radio informing people that American Scientific Research had unearthed chronic withdrawal symptoms about Valium. I listened with interest. Withdrawal symptoms from the drug could last for weeks.

In my experience, the withdrawal symptoms were relentless. Violent sensations throughout my body were particularly severe during the first ten days. I was agitated, combined with migraine headaches, stomach pains that doubled me over, nausea, shakes and chronic anxiety. I didn't know what my body would do next. I could barely live with myself and struggled from one moment to the next to maintain equilibrium. There was little reprieve during the night, and I drifted in and out of sleep.

Just when I thought the worst was over, everything flared up again. In my mind's eye, I can still see myself in the front room, sitting on an armchair, trying to remain in control. I wondered at times if I was going crazy. My immediate concern was not to let anyone see what I was going through. The fear of being readmitted to a psychiatric hospital was overwhelming.

One day, I crawled around on the sitting room floor on all fours like an animal, trying to pull my hair out. Somehow, I managed to pull myself up on the armchair. By then, I knew I needed help. Was there anyone I could trust? The local health nurse popped into my mind.

I heard Tommy's footsteps in the hall, called him and asked him to phone her. When she arrived, I broke down crying. She promised not to tell anyone and reassured me that I wasn't losing my mind. She asserted that the only valid explanation was severe Valium withdrawal because I had come off the drug cold turkey. The *Cambridge Dictionary* explains the term as 'a period of extreme suffering that comes immediately after a person has stopped taking a drug on which they depend'.

The health nurse came every day after that. She encouraged me to eat plenty of fruit, especially grapes and melons, and to drink lots of water to remove the toxins from my body. One day, as she was about to leave, she turned, looked at me and said, 'Every evening, I pray for each of my patients.' I felt reassured.

There were days when I pleaded with her: 'Please, get me Valium.' She encouraged me, saying, 'Breda, you can do it. I promise, though, if you're still this bad when I call tomorrow, I'll get a prescription for you.' When I hadn't improved, she said, 'Look. You've come through another 24 hours without them.

Hang on until this time tomorrow. Please give it another try. I promise that you'll have a good day soon. While there'll likely be a couple of bad days after that, another good day will follow. Then, two or three more until all the bad days are gone. You'll see.'

We had planned to go to America at the end of September to visit Tommy's two sisters, who lived in New York and Florida. The flights were booked. The withdrawal symptoms weren't as bad but were still dragging me down. But on 24 September 1980, we flew out from Shannon Airport for three weeks in New York and Florida.

The worst part of that week was keeping everything bottled up inside. I wasn't myself. Valium withdrawal symptoms continued to be part and parcel of my day. I had no energy. Trying to do the slightest thing took it out of me. Because I couldn't sleep at night, I was played out. I didn't know how to engage in conversations.

During the flight to Tampa, Florida, I brightened up. There was great excitement, but my health continued to drag me down. I did my best to hide that from everyone, but there were telltale signs. One morning, when Tommy suggested bringing the children to the playground, I didn't feel up to it but went. I couldn't even push the swings, and we had to go home early. I went straight to bed but spent the rest of the day beating myself up for being a lousy mother.

Some days, I resorted to having two showers to keep going. Another afternoon, when I tried to hang a few kiddies' clothes on the line, I couldn't. The high temperatures overpowered me. I returned to the house in a terrible state and went straight to bed. When I was with the family, I tried to be friendly, but I was always on the lookout. I didn't want people discussing my health behind my back.

I have happy memories too. In my mind's eye, I can still see Tommy's brother-in-law, a big man, with his arms around our two girls as they sat on each side of his armchair. There was great camaraderie in the house. I couldn't help noticing their love and concern for one another.

The day before we left, we travelled to Disneyland, Orlando. There was excitement and glee written all over the faces of our children.

After disembarking from the plane at Shannon Airport, always a hive of activity, we made our way through the terminal building, collected our car in the car park and drove home. Twenty-four hours later, I was hit by jet lag.

The occurrence disrupts the normal circadian rhythm and can cause psychological and physiological effects such as fatigue, irritability and insomnia. I didn't know that at the time. Had I understood what was happening in my body, I imagine I would have found it easier to cope.

Before lunch the following day, I remember wandering around the house, scared over the severity of what was happening to my body. As well as suffering from the latter stages of Valium withdrawal, I was disorientated, confused and agitated. I didn't know how to cope with the next minute, never mind the next hour.

There was no point in explaining to Tommy when I hadn't the words to clarify what was happening; it was a scary time. Going to bed that night didn't provide the escape I sought. I couldn't sleep.

Regarding Valium withdrawal, I would never recommend coming off the tranquilliser cold turkey. Had I been wiser then, I would have done so gradually.

Chapter 15

MY STRUGGLE TO MOTHER

With my ten-year addiction to Valium behind me, in March 1981, we re-opened for B&B. I was up bright and early every morning, getting the breakfasts ready. There was a significant amount of work involved, with the help of five local girls I cooked the breakfasts, checked the rooms, helped with the washing, drying and ironing, coordinated all our bookings, and did food shopping. Every evening, I prepared four-course dinners, which were open to non-residents.

Predictably, one mid-season morning, I collapsed in an exhausted state. I could not take another step and considered giving up tourism altogether. However, that wasn't an option as we were fully booked out.

While my experiences with psychiatry typically failed to provide the kind of talk therapy I craved, there were a few occasions when I found a place, or person to talk with. Sometimes it helped more than others; getting someone to open up about past trauma in a way that feels safe, rather than overwhelming to them, is a skill in itself.

As I lay in bed resting, my thoughts drifted to something that had been bothering me a lot. The feeling that nobody, not even Tommy, understood where I was coming from was causing me distress.

Tommy didn't fully understand the harmful impact of my history, how severely my health had been affected and knew very little of what I had endured in psychiatric hospitals. I asked him if he would come with me to chat with the local priest. He agreed. The priest welcomed us that night, and I noticed the lovely atmosphere. I felt safe.

I can't recall what we spoke about first, but when I began to talk about childhood memories, how hard my parents had been on me, and how tough my formative years had been, I became visibly upset. When I tried to continue, my body had tensed to such a degree that I had to stop. I know now that opening up needs to happen gradually, in order for a person not to become swamped. I glanced at Tommy and asked, 'Can we go home?' He seemed taken aback but he nodded. We thanked the priest and left. As soon as we got home, I went straight to bed.

The following morning, when I woke, I couldn't move. I felt stuck to the bed. I was still upset over what had happened the night before when even trying to talk about my past had sent me into the horrors. I was ashamed and mortified that both the priest and Tommy had seen me fall apart to the point where I had to get out of the room immediately without a moment's delay. I feared losing control. What must they have thought of me? My behaviour must have looked very odd in their eyes. The more I thought about it the worse I felt.

I saw myself as an insignificant nobody. I didn't count. Everything about me was a disaster. I didn't know how to pull myself together. I was in trouble with my health.

I knew I needed help. From the way I felt inside my head I realised that I wouldn't be able to make it out of the quagmire on my own.

I managed to cook breakfast for our guests. As soon as the rush was over, I drove straight to the Psychiatric Unit in Galway.

The psychiatrist invited me to sit when I entered the small but neat consultation room that held just a table and chair. He was polite, and I felt at ease. He asked me why I had come, and I tried to explain what had happened to me the night before, how I had wanted to share my unresolved past with my husband, but that had been more upsetting than I anticipated, and that I was burnt out emotionally due to pushing myself too hard all summer.

The psychiatrist took notes while I was speaking. I had experienced this before in other psychiatric hospitals. The method always made me uncomfortable. We had no eye contact. What I needed at that moment was someone to listen. To help me understand what had overwhelmed me and suggest how I might cope.

I was assigned a psychiatric diagnosis and prescribed psychotropic medication. These are the notes taken on the day by the attending psychiatrist. And also an added message at a follow-up visit a few weeks later:

Department of Psychiatry
Regional Hospital,
Galway
3 September 1980

Dear Doctor ...,

Your patient came to the Unit of her own accord on the 19 August 1980. Inability to cope, panic attacks, dry mouth, tense muscles, pins and needles, headaches, and no energy seven weeks prior to that. Says that she had worked very hard over the summer and that she was now unable to cope. Feels that part of this may have been due to a marital session with her husband and the local priest. She had to discuss all her childhood and relationships and that it took too much out of her.

On examination, she was mildly depressed, very anxious about her life and work, no thought disorder or psychotic symptoms. Reactive depression in a woman with chronic personality disorder was the diagnosis on this occasion. I suggest a short course of Prothiaden 25mgs., twice daily.

She returned on the 1 September 1980 and claimed of her inability to cope at home – dry mouth, tense muscles, pins and needles, headaches. Denies depression, sleeping normally and no suicidal intentions. Some of these symptoms may be related to the Prothiaden, and because of this I suggested that she discontinue this and with your permission we would like to see her again in two weeks' time.

Yours sincerely,
Doctor …
G.P. Trainee in Psychiatry.

Two weeks later, I signed up for a weekend retreat offered in Athenry by the Redemptorist Order. Within the monastery itself, there was a beautiful atmosphere.

After breakfast, the day began with a prayer period interspersed with hymns. I always came alive during the singing.

Every morning, there was a talk, followed by a quiet time of reflection. The celebration of the Eucharist took place in the evenings, always a truly remarkable and uplifting experience. Throughout the day, there was also an exposition of the Blessed Sacrament for anyone who wanted to spend time in private prayer. I loved the stillness and the sense of peace and connection.

As part of the programme, we were invited to speak to one of the team's priests if something was troubling us. I was impressed by a particular priest's gentle manner, Father Andrew, and arranged to chat with him. His warm welcome made me feel at home right away. I opened up in a way I had never done before, and after the conversation, it was as if a weight had been lifted.

Subsequently, we remained in regular contact. Whenever things got on top of me, I sat down and wrote to him. Doing so gave me a great sense of release, and I could continue with the rest of my day. Father Andrew always replied, and his encouragement gave me the strength to keep going.

Once a month, I travelled to Athenry to see him and chat. On occasion, when I couldn't get a babysitter, I brought our two children, and they were always welcome too. Thus began a friendship that has lasted right up to the present day.

Christmas 1980 came and went, and to my delight I discovered that I was pregnant again in January. The baby was due on 21 September 1981. Apart from severe nausea, everything went well. However, tragedy struck on Friday, 13 August 1981, six weeks before the baby was due.

As I wandered around the sitting room that day, I couldn't feel the baby moving. I tried to reflect on whether I had felt any movement the day before, but my mind went blank. Then I wondered if it was my imagination. Perhaps it was just that the baby had no room to move around anymore.

A couple of hours later, I decided to go to the doctor for a check-up. Try as he would, he could not get the baby's heartbeat. He sent me to the maternity hospital in Galway for an ultrasound scan.

Tommy brought me down. I was shocked when the scan revealed that the baby was dead. To make matters worse, the staff nurse told me I would have to return home and wait until Monday to be induced. Nothing could be done as the hospital staff who did the procedure were off duty for the weekend.

I cannot describe what it was like to live through the rest of that evening and the entire weekend, knowing that I was carrying a dead baby in my womb. At one point, I stood at the kitchen sink, feeling totally unable to carry on with life. At that moment, the words of the well-known hymn 'Nearer, My God, to Thee' crossed my mind. After that, whenever I felt overwhelmed, I sang that hymn silently, which got me by.

> Nearer, my God, to Thee, nearer to Thee.
> E'en though it be a cross that raiseth me;
> Still, all my song shall be nearer, my God, to Thee.
> Though like the wanderer, the sun gone down,
> Darkness be over me, my rest a stone.
> Yet in my dreams I'd be nearer, my God, to Thee.

Early Monday morning, 16 August 1981, Tommy drove me to the maternity hospital in Galway, where I was induced. Tommy was told that my labour could take hours and that it would be best to leave the room and go home. I was too shell-shocked to object.

I don't know how long I was lying in bed before the contractions began. The catering staff dropped food in at mealtimes. Now and then, a nurse peeped around the door, but apart from that, I was left on my own all day. I thought it was because the baby was dead that I had to go through the excruciating labour on my own. The contractions became increasingly unbearable, and I lay squirming in agony.

Later that night, when a nurse came to check how much I had dilated, I was close to giving birth. She hurried to get the midwife. When she arrived, Tommy was allowed in. A medical report noted our baby was born 'around 9.00 p.m.'

The midwife looked towards us both and said, 'It's a boy.' I went numb with grief. As I gazed over, I saw that the younger nurse was agitated before swiping the baby into a blanket and hurriedly leaving the room. Forty-three years later, I can't help thinking if only I could have seen his face. If only I could have held him. I still don't know what happened to that baby or where he was buried.

On 18 August 1981, the gynaecologist, as stated in my file, 'performed an evacuation of retained products'. When I was discharged, I had two small children looking forward to my coming home. That kept me going.

Chapter 16

MY MOTHER

I didn't understand grief around the loss of a baby. I don't think it was widely understood or acknowledged back then; you were expected to just get on with life. I had Fiona and Karen to mind, Tommy had to go back to work the next day, and it was a case of pushing on through. It was very different for mothers then from how it is now.

In the weeks after losing my baby, news came that my mother was battling breast cancer and had to undergo more radiation treatment. She had survived womb cancer five years earlier. We went home to Limerick that weekend for a visit, and as I watched her convalescing in the armchair, something about her made a deep impression. Despite all she had gone through, her quiet resilience, patience and inner strength were a surprise. She told me that her faith had helped her through. She was calm and peaceful. Friendly towards me.

When we left, I did not doubt that she would recover. However, sadly, just before Christmas, she was transferred to St Luke's Hospital in Dublin as the disease had spread. Early January, Tommy and I travelled by train to Dublin to visit her. The roads were treacherous from heavy snow and ice. The drive from Clifden to Galway was horrendous. The carriages jerked abruptly an hour away from Dublin and came to a standstill. The rails were impassable. Then, the heating system on the train failed. Tommy and I stood in the aisle alongside other passengers, shifting from foot to foot to keep warm.

We had nowhere to stay when we arrived in Dublin. Close to midnight, the train pulled into Heuston Station. We found a nearby hotel, the Ashling Hotel, which had one room left. The following morning, after breakfast, we overheard some guests saying there were no buses. That meant a 7km walk to St Luke's Hospital. No roads or footpaths were visible, it was a blanket of snow. Everywhere was cloaked in white. I would never have made it on my own, but Tommy had a wonderful sense of direction. We trudged through and got there.

St Luke's Hospital, Rathgar, Dublin, in the 1980s, was the main hospital in Ireland for cancer treatment. A calming sensation came over me just after I entered the building. The place had an atmosphere that spoke to me of peace. My mother was in a room on her own. Over the next few days, we spent as much time as possible with my mother. The staff couldn't have been more compassionate, helpful and kind. Sadly, at the relatively young age of 58, my mother died peacefully in the hospital on Wednesday, 19 January 1982.

I didn't feel grief. It feels awful to admit, but I was relieved. The worry of trying to relate to her was gone. I still had to attend the funeral. That was hard. The atmosphere in my parents' house compared to Tommy and my family home, felt like walking on eggshells, psychologically unsafe. The tension felt almost unbearable. My relationship with my siblings was very tense, and I felt completely excluded from the conversation. I went through the motions, but during the Mass I turned to Tommy and said, 'You've got to get me out of here.' We left straight after the Mass.

In the weeks after my mother's death, I felt overwhelmed with guilt. What daughter would be relieved that her mother and father had died. I was also troubled by the fact that I felt unable to forgive them. This led to feeling more guilty. All of my life I had grown up with the teaching of the Catholic Church, preaching forgiveness. I was consumed by guilt.

I spoke to our local priest one night at church, telling him how awful I felt that I could not forgive my parents. He looked at me and said, 'That is perfectly normal, understandable, and you have no need to feel guilty. Don't worry one bit more about it.' That was hugely reassuring. He took away the feeling that I was a bad person.

To my joy and delight, I was pregnant again a year later. The due date was 25 September 1983. Thankfully, there were no problems. In mid-August, we attended a neighbour's wedding. We had a wonderful day, and Tommy couldn't get me off the dance floor that night.

At 5 o'clock the following morning, I woke with griping stomach pains, and Tommy phoned for an ambulance to bring me to the maternity hospital. That night, at 8.40 p.m., our baby was born six weeks premature. The next couple of days, life couldn't have been better. Then, an intense pain in my right leg crippled me as I walked down the corridor. A nurse asked the doctor to take a look. He diagnosed thrombophlebitis. A vein in my leg had become inflamed. I needed to remain in hospital for a few more days. The daily treatment involved an injection into my tummy and bed rest.

Twenty-four hours before I was due to go home, the unpredictable happened. I was sitting in the corridor with my baby in my arms when, in total dismay, I watched the life drain out of her toes, feet, legs and up as far as her waist. I thought it was like holding a dead kitten in my arms. I yelled for help. A nurse came, took one look, grabbed the baby and disappeared down the corridor.

Frantic, I rushed to phone Tommy. He reassured me, 'I'll be down soon. Try not to worry.' As I returned to the ward, I noticed a small chapel nearby and went in.

The first thing to catch my eye was a statue of St Gerard Majella, the patron saint of expectant mothers. I knew nothing about him, yet I begged him for help to ensure our baby would be okay. I stayed a few minutes soaking in the peace and then returned to the ward.

After an eternity, I saw a doctor heading towards me. He told me the baby was out of danger and had been given a plasma exchange. Although I didn't know it then, the procedure involves separating and removing the plasma from the blood to remove any abnormal substances circulating in the vital fluid. The red blood cells, white blood cells and platelets are then returned to the body, and the old plasma is replaced with fresh, frozen plasma, a light, amber-coloured liquid.

Two days later, we were discharged. When Tommy and his sister came to collect us, we still had no name for the baby. Her birth had to be registered before we left. My sister-in-law suggested 'Mary'. I shook my head. 'How about Maria?' I loved it. On the way down the corridor with our newborn in my arms, I couldn't have been prouder. Later, what a joy to be home again, introducing the little one to her older sisters.

Over the next fortnight, everything went fine, and the baby was thriving. I only became concerned when I noticed she was sleeping longer than usual. A blood test revealed she had a severe form of anaemia. I froze when the doctor told me that iron could only be given to a baby in tiny doses and that we wouldn't see an improvement for a long time. He suggested that I let her sleep as much as she wanted to.

From then on, whenever Tommy was at work and the girls were in school, the silence in the house was uncanny. To cope, I turned my hand to gardening, where I was close enough to keep an eye on her and get fresh air simultaneously. That's when I got my love for gardening. At the time, the place was bare, just a new bungalow on land typically blasted by sea breezes; the water is visible from our house. I didn't even know I loved gardening, but it was a case of how do you keep yourself sane, when a baby's sleeping around the clock, and it feels like the most unnatural thing for that child to be doing? I didn't realise it at the time, but it was the instinct to get out into nature. There was just a ditch, with nothing on the banks. I remember a neighbour passing on his bike; I didn't know the people in the area, so he was a stranger to me. He looked at me, sized up the situation, and said, 'Ah, easy to know you're a blow in. Do you not realise you're wasting your time? Easy to see you don't know about the sea breezes here.' He made me so determined. I said to myself, *I'm going to prove that man wrong*, and I did. That's what kept me sane during that time.

I can still see myself near the road, at the bottom of a rough grass surrounding the site on which our house was built. In olden times, the field was known as Gáirdín na Meaingeal, the Garden of the Mangels, a vegetable used to feed cows.

Unaware at the time that severe anaemia in babies can result in a delay of developmental milestones, we were heartbroken to see the baby, month after month, lying there on the floor, unable to make any attempt to roll, move around, or crawl. The health nurse told me the left side of her muscles wasn't functioning, and she arranged for a physiotherapist from Galway to work with her once a week. There was still no improvement.

One Sunday, I popped into the sitting room with Maria's dinner in a bowl and placed it on the hearth. She was propped up with cushions on the floor near the window. I glanced at Tommy sitting in the armchair watching television and asked, 'Will you feed her?' He nodded. I turned to go back to the kitchen and was almost at the door when I heard a noise and turned around. I could not believe my eyes. The baby was crawling and heading straight for the bowl of food.

The next day, Monday, the doorbell rang, and I ran to open the front door. I was expecting the physiotherapist and couldn't wait to tell her. She entered the front room as I closed the front door behind her. When she saw Maria crawling around, she looked at me in disbelief and said, 'What's going on? My babies don't get better this fast.' She picked Maria up, hugged her and gave her a check-up. Everything was fine. She turned to me with a broad smile and said, 'I don't need to come here anymore.' I was ecstatic.

In October 1984, I became pregnant again. Those nine months flew by.

On 10 July 1985, I recall lying in bed in the maternity unit, and the lady beside me said, 'What name are you going to call the baby?' 'I haven't a clue.' 'Well, if it's a girl, then, after having so many daughters, you're entitled to call this one after yourself!' I smiled and shook my head, 'There'd be too much confusion.' 'Right, then, how about calling her Breda Ann?' All I could think of was what a beautiful name. Shortly after, I was induced.

Some hours later, when she was born, I felt a deep sense of joy. Throughout her childhood, her aunt, who lived in America, called her 'The Little White Rabbit'. Her long, blonde curls and vivacious character brightened every day. She was five years old when she burst into the kitchen excited and begged me to take the stabilisers off her bike. I shook my head, terrified she'd fall and get hurt. She curled her arms around my leg in such a way I was powerless to move. She looked at me with a beaming smile and said, 'I can, I will, I'm able.' Another evening, when I was feeling down, she ran into the bedroom and said, 'Mammy, I love you to infinity and beyond.'

By Christmas 1985, Tommy and I were expecting another baby. Apart from the usual ups and downs, I was happy and content and even told myself, 'After this baby, I don't mind if I become pregnant again. I'm happy being a mother.' A few days before the baby was due, the gynaecologist arranged for me to be admitted to the hospital the following Tuesday. The Sunday night before that, my husband arrived home from the pub. I was making a baby's cardigan in the kitchen at the knitting machine. I was in flying form. We had a few words, and he went to bed. I stayed up to finish the garment.

Without warning, I was struck by a ferocious pain in my side and a tight sensation across my stomach. I gasped for air. Minutes later, the same thing happened again. I could hardly get out of the chair. When I reached the bedroom, I was crouched over in a shocking state. Tommy was out on the floor in a flash, pulled on some clothes and rushed over to his mother's house to get his two nieces, who were home from England on holiday. Karen, Tommy's niece, came with us to the hospital. Helen stayed behind to mind the children.

I just about managed to get into the car. After multiple pregnancies, instantaneous, rapid, spontaneous contractions can strike from the start of labour. Tommy drove to Clifden at high speed. In the hospital, dazed, I was brought into a side room and put lying on a trolley. I didn't need to hear a nurse saying, 'If you had done your relaxation classes, you wouldn't be in this state now.' Out of character, I shouted at her, 'Get out!' She did.

A doctor arrived, not my own GP, and checked the baby's heartbeat, then turned to my husband and informed him that I couldn't give birth in the hospital because of placenta previa. Tommy replied, 'What if she doesn't make it to Galway?' The doctor threw his arms in the air, shrugged his shoulders and said, 'She has to.' Then, he left the room.

Minutes later, we overheard the ambulance wouldn't start. The battery was dead. The ambulance driver and a female nurse arrived at the room with a wheelchair. I was rushed down the corridor and helped into an estate ambulance. When Karen, Tommy's niece, informed a nurse that she had done her final midwifery exams, she was allowed to come with me. Tommy followed behind in the car.

A retired midwife sat close by, knitting away. She glanced over as my contractions became more forceful but kept on knitting. When two contractions came quickly, and I could hardly breathe, I asked her for help. She patted my arm and said, 'Now, dear, you're okay; you've loads of time.' I knew something was wrong and shouted at Karen, 'Please, look between my legs.' She did. 'Oh my God, we have a baby!'

The nurse rapped on the window and told the driver to stop. Karen couldn't see what she was doing, so she opened the back door of the estate ambulance wide and shouted at Tommy to shine in the car's lights. She asked the nurse for a mucus extractor as the baby wasn't breathing. All kinds of things were flung into the air as she tried to find it.

By now, I was convinced I had yet another dead baby on my hands. Those fears were laid to rest when I heard my baby's cry. Karen said, 'It's a girl!' I was overjoyed. She shouted for a blanket, and the ambulance driver quickly handed her one. She wrapped the baby up snugly before gently passing her over to Tommy through the back door of the estate ambulance, who was standing on the road and looking paler than I'd ever seen him. She needed to attend to me.

Then we heard that the 'flying ambulance' was on its way. I was transferred from one ambulance to another underneath a starry sky. The nurse was lovely. She put the baby in an incubator. A few miles down the road, the driver banged on the window and shouted, 'I need you to turn off the incubator. I can't see the road. The power is affecting the lights.' She jumped up, packed the incubator with towels and turned off the machine. She looked at me and said, 'She'll be fine, don't worry. She's as cosy as could be.'

Upon arrival at the maternity hospital, the baby was taken to a specialist unit to ensure she was okay. My gynaecologist was notified and came to my assistance right away. We were home within a couple of days.

Before we left the hospital two days later, the hospital staff asked us to provide a name so that the baby's birth could be registered. I looked at Tommy, and then asked if we could call her Marguerite after our local health nurse, who had been exceptionally good to me throughout the pregnancy. To this day, I can recall her warm, friendly, caring personality that uplifted me each time she visited our home.

Chapter 17

RECLAIMING MY MIND

By 1990, I knew I needed help to get back on my feet and make sense of my unrelenting distress. We were now parents of five daughters. I was struggling, and I worried about the impact it was having on them. But there's nothing you can do, when you're grovelling on the ground, and you're that sick, the only ambition is to get well. You want to come back for them. But it's out of your control.

Tommy is such a wonderful father. When I was sick, he surrounded the girls with love. One of my daughters told me recently that despite what I went through, she always felt I was there for them when they were growing up. She recalled an incident when she was around 12 or 13, coming into the kitchen and seeing me crying. 'Mum is sick,' Tommy, who came into the kitchen at the same time, said. She went off to her bedroom, and shortly afterwards I followed her, putting my arms around her, giving her the biggest hug. She told me that she would never forget that hug. I would have beaten myself up all my life about being a bad mother, especially to my two older girls. These kinds of memories are so healing to hear. To know that your children might have viewed things differently from how you do.

All my life, I was a timid, withdrawn personality, unable to speak in my own voice. I feared authority in any form. When it came to psychiatry, I perceived doctors as gods and complied with their every instruction.

Yes, I was distressed. My mind, emotions and behaviour were chaotic and disordered. I was extremely hard to live with. Tommy and the children bore the brunt of that. They witnessed shouting matches and heated rows between him and me.

When I remember how childishly I behaved, I want to hang my head in shame. When my emotions overwhelmed me, I resorted to phoney fainting fits. I threw myself on the floor and worked myself into full-blown panic attacks. I had seen my sister having epileptic fits, and I copied her behaviour to get attention.

There were many moments when I felt desperate. Early in our marriage, I recall contacting our GP and pleading with him for a Valium 10 injection. Valium calmed me down and enabled me to pick up on life again. I tried to be a reasonable wife and mother, but there were many times when even that was beyond my reach.

The first years of our marriage were particularly difficult. Tommy had to live with someone who was repeatedly falling apart. He didn't know whether to turn left or right to help me. I can't even begin to imagine what he went through because of me. He had never encountered anyone suffering from depression before. He must have felt utterly helpless, broken, powerless. Those years of our marriage were horrendous.

I recall one occasion when I had been allowed home from St John of God for the weekend. Although I was happy to be in familiar surroundings where I felt safe, I had barely been able to function over those two days. The strain eventually got to me, and I knew I had no choice but to return to the hospital. What must it have been like for Tommy to have to drive his wife to the madhouse on icy, snow-covered roads?

In late spring of 1990 I decided I would see a psychotherapist. I looked up the Yellow Pages and came across the names of two advertised psychotherapists who had private clinics in Galway city. I chanced the first one on the list, unaware that she was also a psychiatrist.

From our first meeting, I felt under pressure to talk about my past. Rather than helping, I couldn't handle the distress that my memories provoked. I found myself completely unable to go about my usual daily routine at home. I recall standing in the bedroom near the radiator, mesmerised as to why I felt this bad. After one session, I called her office to let her know how badly I had been affected by revisiting the past. She refused to engage on the phone and said I had to wait until my next appointment.

Without my knowledge or permission, she contacted my GP. When, in later years, I requested and received my medical file, I found this letter she had written:

Letter to GP: 18 May 1990.

Dear Doctor ...
   I am not going to write a long letter about this lady, as you already have volumes on her. Suffice it to say that I am seeing her on a regular basis, offering supervision and support. The aim of treatment would be to bring about limited changes in her circumstances, so that she has less contact with situations that provoke her difficulties. I would be endeavouring to shift her towards less emphasis on the reconstruction of past events and more emphasis on the analysis of her current behaviour.

> Arising out of your own experiences and involvement with this lady over a number of years, I think you will agree that psychotherapy with these hysterical type personalities gives rise to lots of difficulties, both with the direct and indirect demands that the patients can place on their doctor. At the last visit, Breda had reduced her Melleril to 25mgs at night and in the very near future, I would hope that she will be off this altogether. I will be in touch in due course.
> Best Regards.
> Yours sincerely,
> Doctor …

This letter does not reflect what happened in our sessions. She asked me repeatedly about my past and my feelings about what happened to me. After six sessions, I couldn't take any more. I stopped attending.

A month later, in early June 1990, I was admitted on a voluntary basis to the psychiatric hospital in Ballinasloe, a temporary arrangement until a bed became freed up in Galway Psychiatric Unit. It had been eight years since I had been in a psychiatric hospital.

The room where I was formally admitted was a tightly enclosed space with gaudy pink walls. A psychiatrist asked some questions and took down some details. I was intensely anxious but did everything I could to stay in control. I focused on different objects in the room until, to my immense relief, he spoke. The interview didn't last long. He prescribed Prothiaden 75mg twice daily on top of the Melleril and Gamanil I was already taking.

File report: 12 June 1990. Reported for admission at 11.30 p.m. Tearful and looks depressed. Recurrence of depressive disorder and strong anxiety component. Needs admission. She was cooperative on admission.

Tommy was waiting when I came out of the room. I wanted to tell him I had changed my mind and didn't want to stay. But there was no chance as he was asked to leave immediately. I watched him head down the corridor. Dark memories of other psychiatric institutions flooded my mind.

A tall, clinical staff nurse with a cold no-nonsense demeanour ordered me to follow her. We arrived at a dormitory that contained several single beds. I saw patients turned over on their sides, asleep. Terrified, I got into bed and pulled a heavily starched white sheet over my head.

The feel of the sheets on my skin triggered memories of the three years I had spent in the convent. No one saw my distress because I was well hidden. I was numb all over, curled up in a ball and unable to cry. The added flashbacks to convent life left me in a highly traumatised state. After a while, I drifted off to sleep.

The following morning, the rumpus in the dormitory woke me. I looked on in horror as patients were shouted at and physically dragged out of bed by the nurses. I wondered, did anyone care about these people?

Numb from head to toe, I walked to the day room for breakfast. A dark, oppressive atmosphere hung in the air. Patients seemed lost in a world of their own. After a meagre breakfast, I headed back down the corridor. I met the head staff nurse and asked if I could return to bed. She refused, twice. Her haughty, arrogant behaviour terrified me.

I was angry but also powerless. As has often happened when I've been distressed but unable to express myself, my body did the talking. I started to feel faint. My legs seemed as though they were about to give way beneath me. I had to lean against a wall. I begged once more to be allowed to go to bed. She refused. I turned and went back. A few minutes later, I found the courage to go back and confront her. 'Please, can I tell you I'm not a regular patient here? I'm being transferred to the Psychiatric Unit in Galway later. I want to go back to bed for a while.' She gave in.

After a few hours' sleep, I headed down a dilapidated passageway to the day room. There was nothing to do. The other patients sat in chairs, staring blankly into space. I joined them. The vacant look on their faces unnerved me. How could any human being be reduced to this?

I reached a point where I couldn't stand it any longer. I approached the nurse on duty and said, 'Is there anywhere I can go to do occupational therapy?' She snapped, 'It's unavailable in this part of the hospital.'

All I could do was try and live in the moment. I sat on a chair and began to observe the people around me. No matter where I looked the vacant look on the patients' faces scared me. I couldn't help wondering if they had been so dehumanised and so drugged up that they could no longer communicate. Other patients were shuffling here and there, up and down, as if that was their only occupation in life.

I couldn't stand it. I stood up and wandered down another

passageway that I had spotted to the left of the day room.

The building had been opened in 1833. I glanced into side rooms and bathrooms along the way. Everything to my right and left looked grim. I was appalled at the conditions other patients had to endure. I had to pull back from the filth and stench from the bathrooms.

As I made my way back to the day room, I saw patients who had regressed to such an extent that they had a vacant stare about them and were making unusual noises that unnerved me. One man in particular was making loud, frightening, howling sounds that reminded me of a wild animal. That scared the living daylights out of me, and I couldn't get away fast enough.

Shocked and dazed by all I had seen; lunchtime was a welcome distraction. This meal was also served in the day room. For the rest of the afternoon, the intense boredom crippled me. For something to do, I went up to the day nurse and said, 'Please, can you tell me when I'm due to be transferred?' She looked down her nose at me and in a gruff manner, said, 'Your husband phoned to say he's working on it. I don't have any more information.'

After that, all I could do was hang in there and wait. The hours were endless. To my utter dismay, it was late evening before a minibus arrived. By then, my health was in such a bad place that I had to summon up inner strength that I wasn't sure I had, to appear normal, so that I wouldn't be forced to stay in the hospital.

If the truth were known, I was as weak as water and struggling to stay in touch with reality. After boarding the minibus, I found a place to sit on the left-hand side of the vehicle, a few seats back. I knew it was imperative that I remained in control no matter what. That's why, bang up against the window, I forced myself to gaze out on the streets. What met my eyes seemed surreal. The people, the shops, everything, looked like life on another planet.

When we arrived at the psychiatric unit in Galway, I made doubly sure to keep my composure. I was still shaken and angry at what I had witnessed. But I kept things to myself as I doubted that anyone would believe me.

Psychiatric Unit, Galway

File notes: 13 June 1990
Last night, the patient presented to the unit in a distressed state and had to be held in St Brigid's in Ballinasloe before being transferred here today.

Diagnosis: Depression in a person with chronic personality disorder.

Medication: Continue Melleril 50mgs twice daily and at night. On Gamanil x 2 nights. On Prothiaden 75mgs since yesterday.

For the next couple of days I was confined to bed. There too, I saw other patients being ordered out of bed and stood over until they did so. What gave me a lift now in Galway was that the surroundings were spotlessly clean, and the ward was nice and bright. Still, I had to struggle hard not to let chronic boredom overpower me; it ate into every fibre of my being.

They called it bed rest. It was decided that's what you needed first for a couple of days. You weren't allowed out of the bed apart from going to the bathroom. Just lying there in bed never made sense to me. Eventually you would be allowed out of pyjamas and be given your clothes.

Days were spent with around seven patients in the same ward, always in full view of the nurses' station. It's demoralising to see other human beings in the conditions of my fellow patients. It appalled and frightened me to see people like zombies.

When I was allowed up, there was little to do. Initially, I looked forward to occupational therapy (OT) but became bitterly disappointed when all that was on offer was a small lump of pottery clay handed to each patient. I thought, *This is like giving a child plasticine to play with.* There was a handful of small plastic utensils in the tumbler nearby that were of little use.

There was no open outside area. At the time, the walls were totally blank, no pictures to look at that would occupy your mind. No intellectual stimulation. The majority of your day was spent in the ward in a chair beside the bed.

Apart from OT and a weekly 30-minute relaxation class, the days were long and tedious. To maintain some connection with reality, I walked up and down the corridors. A nurse wrote something I said to her in my chart: 'I don't know whether to sit or stand. I find this hospital stressful. I think I'd be better off at home.'

Nurses report: 14th. June 1990. Constantly putting her hands to her temples, as she says she feels her head is going to burst. Closes her eyes from time to time ...

Another time, I asked the same nurse why there was so little to do and what we did in our pottery classes seemed so childish. She replied, 'I agree with you, but these services are geared towards the elderly and very sick patients.' I walked away thinking, *What about the rest of us?*

I found it increasingly distressing to see fellow patients drugged to the gills. Many walked around like zombies. Others sat all day in chairs, staring into space. It didn't seem right that human beings had been reduced to that.

I found it demoralising that every time I asked the hospital staff for permission to go home, I was refused. That I was a voluntary patient made no difference.

Weekends were the worst. The boredom was crucifying. I remember sitting for hours around a table with other patients and thinking, *Is there not even one doctor who realises the serious damage this type of chronic boredom does to the human brain?*

I often asked if I could leave, but I was always given some reason why that was not possible. Every day, I had to dig deep to find the strength to survive. I was determined not to allow chronic boredom to destroy me.

Over a period of five weeks – from Tuesday 19 June 1990 when I was admitted to Thursday 5 July, the day I was discharged with an appointment to attend the outpatient clinic in three weeks – I was seen by whatever psychiatrist happened to be on duty.

I found it frustrating having to repeat the same information about my past history, over and over again to different doctors. You'd walk into the room, and it would be a complete stranger. Any information you had given to the doctor the previous day was irrelevant, because you had to start all over again as to why you were there. In a two to three week stay, you might see five or six different doctors. It felt as if you weren't getting anywhere. I felt none of the doctors related in a one-to-one conversation; rather, it felt very strict, a list of questions you had to answer, and then they would decide, do we need to up her medication? Do we need to change it? It was all over in five or ten minutes.

Psychiatric Unit, Galway

Medical report: 19th June 1990
Has been having psychoanalysis for past seven weeks. Feels that it was the bringing up of past painful memories of her childhood that has caused her symptoms to deteriorate. Feelings of hopelessness. Feels guilty that she is letting her husband and children down. Agitated. Tense. Tearful. Cooperative. Looks depressed. Speech normal. Rapport established. No evidence psychosis. Insight – 'I am sick, and I need help.'

Diagnosis: Agitated Depression

Medication: Continue Gamanil 70mgs. twice daily. Melleril to 50mgs twice daily and at night.

The boredom in those hospitals was the worst thing. Even if I hadn't been struggling with my mental health, that would have been enough to crack me. One day, it got too much, I felt I couldn't take it anymore. That first time, I chanced it to the hospital chapel.

I made my way down the corridor, all eyes, terrified of being caught and having to stay longer. But I had to get out. My mental health was more important than anyone catching me.

Discreetly, I made my way out a small side door and into the main hospital where I was able to access the small hospital chapel to see if prayer would help. Everything seemed hopeless, but there was a quietness there that I enjoyed, and if only for those few minutes, I was safe. There was a sense of relief, of being able to breathe. I was grasping for something that would help. There was no response, of course there wasn't, so I just sat there for a while, enjoying the peace and quiet, the silence. There was no threat, of seeing things that were appalling to my eyes.

Inevitably, I would have to get back up and go.

There was a coffee shop in the main hospital. I knew nobody in the general hospital would spot me as a psychiatric patient. I had my own clothes. Sometimes I would sit there for a half hour. It was just lovely. A break from the stuff I was witnessing back there. I knew that there were very sick people in that part of the hospital as well, some very feeble, but it was a very different scene to what I was witnessing in the psychiatric wing. This was normal, that wasn't.

Having succeeded in getting to the chapel a couple of times, and not getting satisfaction there, I became braver. Because nobody had spotted me, I decided I was going to go out through the main gate of the hospital.

I managed to get out of the main door of the psychiatric unit without being spotted. I was feeling a bit brazen now. But when you have to do something, you'll do it. I was terrified, because I knew the cost of getting caught. Ordered back into bed and drugged to the hilt, and there for God knows how many extra weeks.

That's how intense the level of boredom was that I was driven to do it.

I made my way out the main doors of the psychiatric unit. Walking down the tarmac, I veered to the right to the main gates of the hospital. It was about a six or seven-minute walk. The main Galway hospital was behind me, to the right was the carpark, to the left was where the nurses stayed. Out of the main gates I crossed the road, turned left, then right, and made my way down to Galway cathedral. This would be far more interesting, with so much to look at. It's actually where Tommy and I got married, because it was halfway between Limerick and Tommy's home. We didn't want to put people out travelling long distances.

There was a little shop in the cathedral that you could browse around. It felt great to be there. In touch with myself again, rather than what I was reduced to in the hospital, where I was silenced and controlled. I was always conscious of time, not to be gone too long in case anyone noticed. Reluctantly, I'd make my way back, not wanting to chance it. There'd be hell to pay if they missed me. I couldn't entirely enjoy the freedom, because of the threat.

I got even braver at other times. Instead of going to the cathedral, I'd go straight, turn right at the traffic lights, and do a loop around the buildings and back up to the hospital. Another day, I came out of the hospital entrance, walked up as far as the Post Office, and went in and wandered around. I needed to see ordinary people living their ordinary lives. Normal business going on.

I never contemplated trying to get home. It would be too dangerous. I was terrified they'd report me to An Garda Síochána, who would then come looking for me. As an escaped inpatient I found it easy to imagine the alarm that would be raised concerning my whereabouts. Even worse, the strict prohibitions that could be imposed on me afterwards, not to mention increased medication to make sure I never rambled out of the ward again.

Each time I managed to find the inner strength to face back into it again. I think I possibly went numb. You know you have to get back there, or you'll be in trouble. I was on autopilot, taking the steps I needed to take to get back in there again. Entering the main hospital was fine but I was always cautious going back into the psychiatric unit. I always made sure there was absolutely nobody around when I did slip in. And I got away with it, every single time.

On one of those walks I decided, *I'm going to have to pretend to be well.* I might have to play that game for a few days, but so what, I'm going to do it. I walked in, made sure I was safe, but as I turned in the main door, and made my way up the corridor towards the psychiatric unit, a psychiatrist recognised me. He said hello and asked how I was, and I replied brightly,

'I'm great, I'm fine, I'm feeling ever so much better.' All bubbly. He said, 'I'm so happy for you.' I thought, *Yay, I pulled it off. Breda keep this up, it's working.* As I made my way back to the ward, I was thrilled, I had managed to pull the wool over his eyes.

Over the next few days, I kept up the pretence. Yet, every time I asked to be discharged the answer was an explicit 'No.' The sheer monotony of every day had a damaging effect on me. Yet again, I couldn't help but wonder whether anyone in the medical field realised that in itself, endless hours of boredom can have devastating effects on the human mind.

One Monday morning, I begged one of the nurses to be allowed home. Bluntly, she replied, 'A team meeting has to take place first before you can be discharged.' I inquired, 'When is that meeting scheduled?' She responded, 'The week after next.' I was shocked. How could I be expected to wait that long? I was already at my wits' end.

Over the next couple of weeks, I had to find inner resources that I didn't know I had in order to cope. After an endless wait, when the team meeting did occur, I was surprised to hear that I could attend. However, surrounded by a circle of medical personnel, I felt invisible and when I was addressed, I chose my words carefully. The discussion went in my favour, and I was to be discharged as an outpatient, with immediate effect.

Discharge summary: 5th July 1990

Reason for Admission: The patient has felt depressed, tense, and anxious for years, but this has worsened for the last six weeks. She also complained of poor sleep and early morning wakening. She was unable to cope with her housework, due to loss of energy.

Final Diagnosis: Depressive illness

Medication: Melleril 50mgs. twice daily and at night. Gamanil 70mgs. twice daily.

Chapter 18

SICK OF BEING SICK

When I returned home, I had a severe tremor throughout my body. I found it impossible to steady my hand enough to write, and it was noticeable enough that my daughter pointed it out. I made an outpatient appointment with the psychiatric department. When Tommy and I arrived at the hospital, we were led into a small consulting room by a psychiatric registrar. When I told her what the medication was doing to me, she wouldn't hear of it. Tommy backed me. She ignored him. She looked at me with an air of authority and said, 'You have Parkinson's disease.' I was shocked. Tommy couldn't fathom it either. With nothing left to say, we turned and went home.

I found two reports in my file, written by the same doctor on the same day.

> **File notes:** 26th July 1990. I saw this woman at the outpatient clinic today. Her present medication is Modecate 12.6mgs. intramuscular every three weeks, Melleril 25mgs. at night and Cytrin, one twice daily. She had no complaints. She has a known history of Parkinson's disease. Her sleep, appetite and energy were good. Her interest was also good. She denied any psychotic symptoms. I plan to review her again in two months.

I had never once in 20 years had any doctor refer to Parkinson's disease.

Letter to GP: 26th July 1990

I saw this patient at the outpatient clinic today. Her present medication was Gamanil, one in the morning and at night, and Melleril 50mgs. in the morning and 50mgs. at night. She felt overall improved but still complained that she suffered from depression and her mood particularly being worse in the morning.

She found it difficult to develop an interest, and her energy was poor. Her appetite was good, and her sleep has much improved. She found her husband very supportive in her complaints. She had no death wish or suicidal ideation. She was very pleasant and well-dressed, and her mood was depressed. I plan to decrease her Melleril to 25mgs. in the morning, and 50mgs. at night and increased her Gamanil to 70mgs in the morning and 140mgs at night. I plan to review this again in two weeks.

No mention of Parkinson's disease in the second note, but equally no reference to or explanation for my reason for asking for an appointment.

I returned to see the consultant psychiatrist two weeks later, but nothing had changed. I was under his care for five years. When I returned for a second follow-up appointment after a month, he wrote the following:

> **File notes:** 13 February 1991. Terrible month. Sleeps through the night. Concentration fair. Works with effort.

> Reduced interest. No energy. Tryptizol 50mgs twice daily. 100mgs at night. Lithium 300mgs, morning and night. Melleril 25mgs at night. To attend Clifden Support Centre twice weekly. Feels she is not back completely to her pre-morbid level. Mood fluctuates, worse in the morning. Coping better with housework; feels better able to make an effort.

He attributed any improvement to psychotropic drugs. I saw it differently. Since I was a child, I had to fight hard to get through each day despite debilitating body sensations. I had endured beatings and peer rejection and had been forced to work long hours. By this stage of my life, I knew how to survive.

What helped me most while under psychiatric care was the time I spent in nature. From the days spent with my father as a child, gardening, to being outdoors in our home in Connemara, nature had always been a source of calm. I had taken to working with Tommy in the bog near our home, turning and footing turf, a carrycot in tow while the baby slept. I spent the summer months in the field below our house, helping my father-in-law to shake and save the hay manually. I loved the fresh air and in the evenings the satisfaction of a job well done.

I wanted to challenge this consultant psychiatrist. But I remained mute for fear I would be ridiculed, have my meds increased, or be readmitted to hospital. There were days when I did not want to attend an appointment, but I was afraid he'd issue a detention order if I didn't show up. Refusing to go along with what he was instructing simply did not seem like an option.

Altogether, I was 23 years under the care of the psychiatric system. I was prescribed Valium, Parstelin, Mogadon, Melleril, Tryptizol, Prothiaden, Camcolit, Lithium, Prozac, and Seroxat.

In the early spring of 1995, at yet another appointment, this same consultant psychiatrist looked up at me from his desk and said, 'There are four families of antidepressant drugs. I have tried you on each one, and none has worked. I'm now going to add Optimax.'

He had an additional air of confidence about him that day as he wrote in my file, insisting that the new combination would work. I was alarmed when he informed me that, 'In some cases, Optimax has badly affected a person's leg muscles. However, that is unlikely to happen to you.'

Why was I being prescribed such a dangerous drug? Despite his reassurances, how would that affect me? When I got outside the main door of the psychiatric unit, I stood motionless at the entrance for ten minutes. *What if the psychiatrists themselves don't know what's wrong with me? If anyone could see what it's like to try and live inside my body, surely I would be offered more support,* I thought.

What was supportive was attending the Clifden Support Centre twice a week. I was happy there. The staff were caring, and I got on well with everyone. In particular, I loved the pottery classes. The teacher was a ceramic artist, and with her help, I made some pieces I have kept to this day.

After three weeks of taking Optimax, I mentioned to the nurse in charge that I was a little worried about taking this drug as it didn't seem to be working. If anything, my mood felt worse. 'Don't worry,' he replied. 'Give it time; it will work.' It didn't.

Letter from GP to the Community Welfare Officer:
28 March 1995

Dear Mr ...

This is to inform you that Mrs Breda O'Toole is currently on Optimax (Tryptophan). A medication which was recently commenced by Doctor ..., consultant psychiatrist UCHG. This drug is not available on the GMS, and Mrs O'Toole is unable to pay for it herself. We would appreciate your consideration on the matter.

Yours sincerely

Doctor ...

Monday morning of Holy Week, 10 April 1995, I got up and struggled to get to the kitchen and make a cup of tea. I was in a terrible state, things were worse than ever. Unable to make it across the room, I grabbed a stool to sit down. *What's going on here?* I asked myself. I didn't know about mindfulness at the time, but what happened next was a body scan. I thought, *That's depression over there. I know what that feels like. This is something totally different.* An image formed in my mind almost like a mesh of wires; I could almost see the criss-cross interaction of all the drugs. It was just an image that came into my mind, but it made sense to me. *All those drugs I'm on, that's what this is. That's why I can't get over to put on the kettle.*

I had a sudden moment of clear understanding. *This is not about depression. What I'm experiencing now is the interaction of the 15 tablets a day I'm on. They're not helping; they're driving me crazy.* I wanted to try to make a change.

I phoned the psychiatric unit and made an appointment to see the consultant psychiatrist the following day. After a three-hour wait, we were told he was unavailable and that his registrar would see us instead.

She guided us into a small, familiar-looking consulting room. We remained standing while she flipped through my file. All of a sudden, alarmed by what she had read, she said, 'Breda, you need counselling for sexual abuse. I need to discuss this with your consultant.'

I was relieved that, finally, we could begin to address the root cause of my health problems. When she went next door to report to the consultant whose care I was under, we heard him shouting her down. She emerged from the room and said, 'He won't agree to counselling but has agreed to reduce your medication a little.' We thanked her and went home.

That Thursday, I was booked to play the organ for that night's service and run the choir. I felt dreadful but didn't want to let anyone down. As I made my way up to the altar, a woman I know stopped me. 'Breda are you okay? You don't look well.' I said, 'No I'm not,' and then I just carried on, slightly in a world of my own.

At that time – it doesn't happen now – there used to be what was called the exposition of the Blessed Sacrament, where the Sacred Host would be on the altar, and you could go in and pray. There would be beautiful flowers and a fabulous atmosphere in the quietness of the night. I decided I would go home and get a cup of tea, and then come back to the church to pray. It's not that I had great faith, but I was desperate. This was the one and only person I could think of who might be able to help, whoever or whatever He was; I couldn't see Him, but I knew He existed somehow.

I left Tommy at home with the kids and drove to the church in a kind of mental fog. Once back at the church, I knelt on the altar step for 40 minutes, repeating over and over, 'Please give me back my health. Please give me back my health.' It was like a mantra. I was barely able to get up again, but eventually I made my way out and went home.

The following morning, the phone rang. Still feeling dreadful, I stumbled across the kitchen to pick up the receiver. I was surprised to hear it was the Jesuit priest who had facilitated the parenting course in Galway, Father Paul: vivacious, full of life, enthusiastic, very alive. By this stage we had become good friends; he knew me very well.

We talked, and it was clear to Father Paul how unwell and low I was. After a few minutes, Paul said forcefully, 'Breda, take back control of your life.' I asked him, 'Paul, I'm sorry, what do you mean by that?' I could hear his disbelief on the other end of the phone. I'd never heard him speaking that firmly to me. This might seem unbelievable, but I had not a clue what that man meant. Not a clue.

I know this might seem strange, or hard to understand, but not doing what the psychiatrists said had never occurred to me until this moment. It was the times that were in it. There was a similar thing going on with the church. The power of those two institutions. What they said went. Nobody questioned that.

'Can you not see it?' Paul replied that day on the phone. 'You've handed control of your life over to the psychiatrists. From what I've seen over recent months, they've made a bloody disastrous job of it.' He stunned me. I went silent. After I put down the phone, something just rose up in me, and I thought, *That's it.* I decided I would get myself off all medication. They talk nowadays about wake-up calls. That's the only way I can describe it now. I realised Paul was right, and then my determination fired up.

I knew only too well what coming off Valium cold turkey had done to me. This time, I promised myself that I would do so gradually.

I was taking Seroxat, 40mg in the morning; Tryptizol, 50mg in the morning and 100mg at night; Camcolit, 500mg in the morning and 750mg at night; Eltroxin, 100mg in the morning; and Optimax, 1g in the morning and 1g at night. Fifteen tablets a day.

I was on thyroid medication Eltroxin to counter the effects of the psychotropic drugs on my thyroid. I was advised by my GP that it was a dangerous drug to come off without supervision. He recommended I do so by reducing my intake of one tablet a day to half a tablet for a couple of weeks before coming off it altogether.

I had no withdrawal symptoms. I was very careful to gradually reduce the drugs I was on. I wanted to act responsibly. I went to my GP once a week to have a blood test done to make sure there were no adverse effects. Each of the blood tests came back normal. That gave me a great boost.

My weight had dropped from 12½ stone to 10½ stone without walking or going on a diet. My severe body tremor disappeared. I am now more than 30 years medication-free.

My health improved, and people began to remark on how

well I looked. I took the summer to get myself off all medication. As the weeks passed, I was conscious of the psychiatrist under whose care I had been for the past five years not knowing one single thing about this. I like being upfront with people. I wanted to be honest with him. I made an appointment to go and see him that October. I wasn't nervous. I was my own person now. I was determined. But I wanted him to know. I don't like giving anyone false impressions.

When I entered his office, he commented, 'I have never seen you looking so well.' I sat on the chair and told him I had weaned myself off all medication. There was silence in the room.

To ease the tension between us, I said, 'I got sick of being sick.' He replied, 'It can happen like that sometimes.' Even though I had been successful in getting myself off all medication, I knew I still needed support. I said, 'In your professional capacity, could you please recommend a good therapist?' He replied, 'You don't need counselling. You're more than well able to cope with anything.'

Despite the compliment, I had my doubts. There was nothing left to say. I thanked him and got up to leave. He stood up, too, and we shook hands. As I touched the door handle to let myself out, I heard a loud, booming voice behind me say, 'But, I'm warning you to stay on Lithium.' I froze. But in that same moment, I decided that I knew what I was doing, and I wouldn't back down. I would never again allow anyone to dictate to me.

The following week, I returned to the local support centre in Clifden. I sat at the table and had just settled in to do more pottery when the nurse in the centre came over. He bent down and whispered gently, kindly, that he needed to talk to me and asked if I could come to his office. I was surprised. Nothing like that had ever happened to me before.

He invited me to sit down. 'Breda. I'm sorry, but I've received orders from Galway not to let you attend the support centre. The consultant psychiatrist has forbidden it and has ordered me not to let you in unless you agree to take Lithium. Breda, he is livid with you because you've stopped taking your medication. He's saying it's proof you're manic.' That sounded incredible to me. As upsetting as it was to be told I could no longer attend the centre, I never considered agreeing to these terms. I knew the destruction those drugs had caused my body. And I knew the fight I'd had on my hands to get off them.

I left the support centre shocked to the core. I felt numb as I walked into town, the world around me feeling more unreal with every step I took.

That consultant psychiatrist's view was summarised in a letter he wrote to a neurologist whom I attended for ongoing pain two years later:

Letter to neurologist: 9 September 1997

Dear Doctor ...

Many thanks for your request on the above. In 1990, she was first referred to me, and at that stage, she was admitted in June with symptoms of a depressive illness. (See enclosed discharge summary.) At that time, she was prescribed Gamanil 70mgs twice daily and Melleril 50mgs. three times daily and at night.

Subsequently, she attended me regularly with symptoms of a chronic depressive nature for which she was prescribed Lithium and various antidepressants. Her condition gradually improved, but she required significant doses of antidepressants. For instance, on 7 March 1994, she was taking Faverin 50mgs in the morning, Tryptizol 50mgs in the morning and 100mg at night. Camcolit 500mgs in the morning and 750mgs at night, Lithium and Eltroxin 100mg. daily.

She showed a gradual improvement from there on, but with a recurrence of her depression in April 1995, I switched her from Faverin to Seroxat 40mgs in the morning and put her on Optimax, 1 gram in the morning and at night.

I believe her diagnosis to be Bipolar Affective Disorder. She was well-stabilised on Lithium when last seen.

Yours sincerely,

I do not believe I suffered from bipolar affective disorder. I resent that I had to take Lithium for five years, from 1991 to 1995.

During my twenties, thirties and forties, I was indeed a very vulnerable person. I see this now. However, in my mid-forties, I began to see that psychiatry was making things worse, and I gradually removed myself from those services. Since November 1995, I've grown and matured, and through therapy I have developed a much stronger sense of myself.

Part Three:

LOVING THE STRANGER
WHO WAS MYSELF

Chapter 19

MY 'ONE GOOD ADULT'

By now, my relationship with Tommy was a disaster. He didn't know what to make of me. I was wrapped up in a world of my own that was both terrifying and impossible to live with. I was barely ticking over.

It pained me that he didn't understand what I was going through. I was frustrated and angry, and I had no one to turn to. Even access to the support centre in Clifden had been taken away from me by the psychiatrist in Galway because I had weaned myself off all medication. I ended up completely closed in on myself.

I was the one not talking to Tommy; I didn't know how and that created its own tensions. We just kept brushing past one another. I felt we were drifting apart. That scared the life out of me. The strain and the tension in the house were palpable. I was trying badly to get by but was in a bad way.

My friend Father Andrew, whose retreat and events I used to attend in Athenry rang me one day. One of the first people I had opened up to, he had become, and remains, a good friend. Even though, in my childhood especially, the Catholic Church was an institution, not unlike psychiatry, which was powerful and intimidating, and by which I felt silenced, in my adult life I have been helped along the way by several members of the clergy to whom I am grateful.

After I picked up the phone, I broke down in floods of tears, unable to speak. He said, 'Breda, what's wrong?' And I said, 'My marriage is falling apart.'

Almost in the same tone as Paul, Andrew said bluntly, 'Breda, for God's sake will you get yourself to David.' I didn't know who he was talking about. He explained that David was a clinical psychologist specialising in psychotherapy.

The reality of it is I probably wouldn't be alive today without David.

We all need understanding and support to get to the root of persistent emotional and interpersonal distress. In spite of my frequent engagements with both public and private mental health services over 20 years, I never found someone to help me come to terms with what was happening in my life. Until I met David – someone who believed in me and worked with me for an extended period.

I rang on a Wednesday, and he saw me on the Friday. David was different from other professionals I had met. He wasn't an intimidating presence; he was a very peaceful presence. I felt safe right away with him. He warmly greeted me and invited me to sit down. Then he said to me, 'What is it I can do for you?' I was dumbfounded. Nobody had ever asked me that before. He wasn't seeing me as sick. It was so different to everything I had experienced. I went blank. I had never been asked a question like that before, and I didn't know what to say.

I told him I just want to get my health back. He listened as I tried to describe what I'd been through. He looked at me, with care but also a sense of seriousness, and he said, 'Are you willing to go through more blood, sweat and tears?' I nodded and said, 'Yes.' I would have done anything to get well again. I was determined to work with him no matter what it took.

I met him the following week in Galway city.

MY 'ONE GOOD ADULT'

He had suggested we meet again, and that Tommy come with me for the first session. I agreed even though I felt uncomfortable with the idea. In hindsight that was a disaster, and I should have just gone with my gut and gone to see him on my own.

On the way to the appointment the following week in Galway, I insisted on driving – it was the only way I felt I had control. I was in a desperate state, barely hanging in there. Frightening sensations soared through my body. I felt severely numb, and my head was rock solid. I felt sick to my stomach. I had no words to explain this to Tommy. He didn't know what was going on. There was a stone wall tension between us. And yet my heart was crying out for Tommy to understand. For someone to understand. From the word go, I knew that David got me. I didn't have to explain, he just understood.

The drive down was a nightmare. The only way I could cope was listening to a Charlie Landsborough (a British singer) CD on repeat; it was my way of totally blocking out. I must have driven Tommy demented. When we arrived at David's office, I was a bag of nerves. David, totally composed as always, greeted us with a warm welcome. It would do you good to be in his presence, he had such an aura of peace. It was a bright, spacious room that helped me to feel I was in a safe place. He invited us to sit and said a few kind words to me before turning to Tommy.

I sat there passively as if I had lost my voice. I saw David nodding at Tommy and agreeing with him. Seeing two men chatting about me and agreeing with each other was unnerving and frustrating. All I could think was, *I don't stand a chance here*. I panicked. After holding myself together for several minutes, I jumped up and ran out of the room. David didn't come after me. He gave me space to recover in my own good time. I was grateful for that.

I sat on a step and bawled my eyes out. Tommy told me afterwards that he had wanted to come out after me, but David said, 'No, let her be.' He knew I would recover in my own time.

He was right. After about ten minutes, I found the courage to return. I opened the door and quietly took my seat. David gave me a kind, reassuring look, but didn't say a word about what had happened. I wasn't confronted or asked to explain myself. Again, I knew I was in a secure place, where I was understood.

I don't remember what we talked about afterwards, but I left that session feeling I was in safe hands. He asked me if I would like to see him again the following week; there was no pushiness, it was all up to me. I saw him on my own the following week.

As the weeks passed, I began to look forward to my sessions with David. He listened and took me seriously. I felt he related to me as an equal, with respect. Finally, I had found someone with whom it was safe to face reality. There was something totally different in his approach to me. I was in awe of the man.

Early on in our sessions, he gave me a handout outlining the Ten Cognitive Errors.* I took it home to read, and realised I saw myself in every error on the list:

---

* Adapted from Table 3-1 in *Feeling Good, The New Mood Therapy* by David D. Burns, MD. (William Morrow and Company, Inc., 1980; New American Library, 1981.)

1. **All-Or-Nothing Thinking:** You see things in black-or-white categories. If your performance falls short of perfect, you see yourself as a failure. This type of thinking causes you to fear any mistake. Absolute perfectionism does not exist in this world, and this error sets you up to repeatedly experience the feeling of total failure.
2. **Overgeneralisation:** You see a single adverse event as a never-ending pattern of defeat. For example, you're late for an appointment or make a mistake and tell yourself, 'I'm always doing that.' This type of thinking causes hopelessness as the past, present and future are distorted into a never-ending pattern of failure.
3. **Mental Filter:** You pick out a single negative detail and dwell on it exclusively, allowing one person to pull you down as if they have exclusive insight into your limitations while ignoring your beautiful strengths.
4. **Disqualifying the Positives:** You reject positive experiences by insisting they 'don't count' for some reason.
5. **Jumping to Conclusions:** You interpret things negatively when no definite facts support your conclusion. There are two ways this can happen. *Mind Reading:* You insistently conclude that someone is reacting negatively to you without checking it out. You jump to a conclusion about what other people are thinking. *The Fortune Telling Error:* You anticipate that things will turn out badly. For example, before a meeting, you repeatedly tell yourself, 'I'm going to blow it. My mind will go blank. I'll make a fool of myself.'
6. **Magnification (Catastrophising) or Minimisation:** You exaggerate the importance of your mistakes or problems or

inappropriately shrink the significance of your desirable qualities. Conversely, you may magnify the importance of someone else's achievements and minimise your own. This is also called the 'Binocular Trick'.

7. **Emotional Reasoning:** You assume that your negative emotions reflect how things are. This kind of reasoning is misleading because your feelings reflect your thoughts and beliefs. If they are distorted or twisted, your emotions are not valid. One side effect of emotional reasoning is procrastination, putting off what can be done today until tomorrow.

8. **Should Statements:** You try to motivate yourself to do better with 'should' and 'shouldn't'. These words pressure you because of the unnecessary expectations you have to live up to. When you don't quite achieve the target you have set for yourself, you feel guilty and ashamed. When other people's performance exceeds your expectations, you feel resentful and bitter.

9. **Labelling:** Instead of saying, 'I made a mistake,' you attach a negative label to yourself. Labelling yourself or others is quite destructive because you tend to feel the problem is with a person's defective 'character' or 'essence' instead of with their behaviour. When you label other people, you will always expect that person to behave negatively. This makes you feel angry and hostile towards the other person.

10. **Personalisation:** You blame yourself for an event you were not entirely responsible for. This thinking error will make you feel hugely guilty, like unnecessary expectations and the use of the words 'should', 'ought', and 'have to'.

It was as if a whole new fascinating world was opening up to me. I felt he saw only the positive qualities in me, which helped me deal with my own pessimistic thinking.

One handout he gave me showed me how our thoughts affect our mood:

> When you are experiencing a blue mood, the chances are that you are telling yourself you are inherently inadequate or just plain 'no good'. You become convinced that you are worthless.
>
> If you believe such thoughts, you experience a severe emotional reaction of despair and self-hatred. You may become inactive and paralysed, afraid and unwilling to participate in the normal flow of life. You may even wonder if you'd be better off dead.
>
> Rotten, miserable internal states do not prove that you are a horrible, worthless person, merely that you think you are.
>
> Recognising the negative emotional and behavioural consequences of our harsh thinking is a significant achievement. In time, we can learn to see that our thoughts are incorrect and unrealistic.
>
> Human life is an ongoing process involving a constantly changing physical body and rapidly changing thoughts, feelings, and behaviours. Your life, therefore, is an evolving experience, a continual flow. You are not a thing, so any label is constricting, highly inaccurate, and global. Abstract tags such as 'worthless' or 'inferior' communicate nothing and mean nothing.

Your feelings do not determine your worth, nor do your thoughts or behaviours. Some may be positive, creative and enhancing; most are neutral. Others may be irrational, self-defeating, and maladaptive. The more we notice these thoughts filling our minds and catching them before they take hold, the greater our chance of not buying into them. This is not easy. Overcoming our negative thinking habits requires consistent practice and an attitude of kindness towards ourselves.

David frequently told me a story to communicate a point he wanted to make. One that has stayed with me was about a flock of birds that had to flee their nests because an intense fire raged in the forest. It seemed as if everything was lost. But where the birds ended up was indescribably more beautiful. The large tree they found to build their nests was even more striking and beyond anything they could have hoped for.

He explained how a gorse fire is necessary before new growth can emerge. Storms help clear the atmosphere to create something new. Slowly, I began to see my disturbing episodes as having within them an opportunity for me to grow.

I would see David as his client for 23 years. Even after he retired, he continued to coach me. For the first two years of therapy with David, the panic attacks were day after day after day. My head was in such a frenzy. But I felt so safe with him; I would grab the pen and paper again and write honestly about what I was thinking and feeling. It was my way of getting some sort of control over what was happening to my body, because the worst part of a panic attack is the feeling that you have lost control.

I wrote down exactly what was happening to my body at the time. For example, that I was shaking all over, that I was completely unable to function, that I was gasping for breath and my body was going crazy. It didn't take much to imagine that if anyone saw me in that state I'd be rushed to a psychiatric hospital.

But I knew from similar episodes in the past that my body would eventually calm down. Though shaken by the experience, I was always able to continue with my day. Writing down what was happening saved me from losing my head. My writing might be a scrawl by the end, but I got it out.

In part, I think the panic attacks were probably because of the work David and I were doing. It wasn't David who upset me; it was facing extremely painful issues in my life that I had never faced – or been allowed to face – up to that point. Meeting oneself in therapy isn't easy at the best of times. But choosing to open sealed-off memories of trauma is intensely distressing.

Therapy is a safe space where we can express our emotions. It takes time and requires patience and courage. Therapy gradually uncovers our wounds and scars and stirs emotions that can shake us to the core. For stretches of time, we may feel intensely vulnerable and wonder what the point is. We may imagine therapy is making us worse rather than better. We may feel we are falling apart when, in truth, we are coming together.

David created a safe space, lighting a path through the darkness. It felt like having an ally as I worked my way through everything that had been holding me back from living my life. There were many times during a therapy session when I would go into a negative spin about the past and my body would become tense. Head down, unable to look my therapist in the eye, I can easily recall how uptight I used to become. I can still see myself trying to get out the words I wanted to say while at the same time struggling with an upsurge of painful emotions and sensations. These occasions took so much out of me I was frightened of losing control. I would also become highly defensive.

When Tommy acted in a way I didn't like – for example, what I perceived as ordering me to do something instead of asking me in a nice tone of voice – I would retaliate strongly and give out hell. Inevitably, a row would break out.

When I discussed this with the therapist, I blamed Tommy high up and low down. I wasn't the problem, he was.

In his compassionate way, time and time again over many years, David would reassure me, 'Breda, the past is gone. It doesn't exist. All that matters is the present.' And I would feel back in the driver's seat, with a new sense of hope and a happier outlook towards life.

Along the way, it was clear at times that my body wasn't right. I started seeing David in November 1995. I had weaned myself off all medication that summer. But I was still a very traumatised person. I had left behind 23 years of psychotropic drugs. There was no way my body could have repaired itself in that short time. I was still experiencing a mix of my anxiety around life, my ability or inability to cope, anxiety about relationships at home with my family, and the sheer effort I had to put into getting through each day. My body was just in high doh. At the time, I still didn't know that what I was experiencing were panic attacks. But I knew I could not afford to let one other human see me in that state, or I would be shifted back into a psychiatric hospital. I worried that if Tommy saw me in that state, he would get on to the GP and I would be put back in hospital. It was a secretive world that I was living in.

David encouraged me to write down my feelings between sessions – there's only so much you can talk about in an hour. At home, there were times when difficult sensations in my body were so intense that I felt entirely overwhelmed, as if I couldn't continue with life. My mind was frenzied. Simply going to the sink to wash a cup felt like too much.

In those moments, I would grab a sheet of paper, sit down and describe exactly what was happening to me. Rather than hiding what I felt out of shame, I found a way of communicating my reactions to everyday challenges to another human being and of telling them about my past. Writing it didn't take as much out of me as talking about it face to face sometimes did. With a pen and paper, you're alone with yourself.

I didn't realise it at the time but what I was engaged in was journalling. I found it very healing, a form of self-soothing. I would sit in the armchair in our front room, facing the big wide window looking out on the lake: a safe space in our own home. It was like the pen had a life of its own at times. I always felt better, and reenergised afterwards, able to continue with the rest of my day.

At one point, it felt too much, and I told David I had had enough. I wanted out of life. He didn't overreact. He listened, and I knew he heard what I was saying. I left his room that day in tears but also deeply grateful he hadn't rushed me off to a psychiatric hospital. I always found his composure, unconditional acceptance and caring attitude comforting.

Chapter 20

LEARNING TO BE A MOTHER

Thanks to David's encouragement, I began to risk small changes in my life. For example, I'd always believed that once I'd prepared dinner, my duty to the family was done. While everyone else ate at the table, I sat beside the range in the kitchen and ate my dinner alone. I saw nothing wrong with that until we considered the importance of sharing a meal with others and what I was missing by not sitting with the family. I started to sit with my family at mealtimes and discovered how enriching it can be to share meals.

When I first started seeing David in 1995, there was tension in our house. I was sick, and I found it hard to relate to the girls beyond providing for their physical needs. I didn't even know that there was such a thing as emotional needs. There was always food when they came home, their clothes were always looked after, but I was sometimes unable to express my love for them beyond that.

As the girls got older, one of my biggest concerns was improving our relationships at home. We now had five daughters with a five-year gap between the eldest two and the younger three. But I was persistently on edge within myself.

During the teenage years, rows were frequent and they rattled me. Hearing the three younger ones fighting in the front room while I was preparing dinner, I'd rush in, all hot and bothered, look at the older of the three and say, 'What's going on? Why are you upsetting everyone?' which always made things worse.

Tommy tried to reassure me repeatedly, 'It's just a stage they're going through; it will pass.' Years later, in a light-hearted way, that same daughter said, 'Mum if you had only left us alone, we would have sorted it out between ourselves.'

One day in a session, after another row with Tommy, David looked at me and said, 'Breda, what I would suggest is, all that, that's the past, it's gone. This is the present. Try now to create a haven of love in your home. It just takes one person. Love yourself first. And then loving others will be a cinch.' At the time, I didn't know what he meant. But in the weeks after, moment by moment, I just tried to have a loving response to whatever was happening around me. If the kids came to me, I took that moment and tried to think of creating a haven of love. And it worked.

My tendency at the time was to cut my children short if they came to me with a question or were nagging me about something or other. The quicker I could get rid of them the better. I found the repetitive nature of their questions annoying.

I decided to try and change that. I began to smile when they came to me instead of being grumpy. I did my utmost to be more present to them. I put in the extra effort it takes to listen to what they were saying, even when it went against the grain. I always felt better for it afterwards and the children ran off happy and content.

Over time, I learned to wait until things had quietened before trying to sort out difficulties when feelings were running high. My therapist pointed out that 'Children usually express their anger only if their home environment feels safe enough to do so.' I found his words reassuring. He also reminded me that as teenagers get older, they also become more settled.

I left his office that day feeling more hopeful. Later, as Tommy and I cleaned up after dinner, I said, 'I feel so bad over the number of times I've said to Maria that because she's older, she should know better.' Tommy replied, 'All you need to do is not say it anymore.'

Of course, Tommy and I didn't always agree. When one of the younger children asked her older sister for a spoon, she was refused. Tommy, busy at the sink washing dishes, said, 'When your sister asks you for a spoon, you should give it to her.' I rushed to her defence, saying, 'She was already doing something, let the child get the spoon for herself.' This caused a heated row between the two of us. I refused to back down. There were consequences. I became so distressed that Tommy never got to check the cows that evening. I was too upset to go to a concert I had been looking forward to for weeks.

I believed I was right to speak up for our eldest daughter, who always helped others. It was just that once that she said no. My therapist, David, taught me that a united front is important because children get confused when they hear mixed messages. Arguments can unnerve them when they don't understand what's happening. I learned that it's wise to remain silent and discuss disagreements later, and I've tried to do this ever since.

The next evening, Tommy and I walked to the beach near our home. More than anything else, I wanted to be upfront with him, but I struggled to be open. That meant going outside my comfort zone. I swallowed my pride and told him that during my therapy session that day I had told David about the row the night before to check whether or not I had been right to stick up for Fiona, my eldest daughter. David agreed with Tommy! To admit that to him took guts. It was a humbling experience. But, somehow, I did, and he heard me. The heart-to-heart conversation that followed brought us closer.

I still had to learn how to hug my children. I was never hugged as a child, and for years I didn't see its relevance. I thought I was doing a good enough job once I was providing for my children's physical needs. It was only when I saw Tommy and his family hugging not just our children but each other that I began to wonder why I wasn't able to do the same.

It took me a while to unfreeze my arms and attempt to hug. I took small steps at first by hugging our smaller children now and then. It took me longer with the older girls. I was afraid they would think me strange, but they soon liked it as much as I did. Today, being able to hug my children and allowing myself to feel their love's warmth is one of my greatest joys.

On occasion, I was still stuck in the patterns and behaviours I had learned as a child. One evening, about ten minutes before Tommy was due home from work, overpowering sensations took over my body. In a heightened state of panic, I dashed around the house frantically, trying to clean the place so that it was in order for him. Not that he expected it from me, but I had learned as a child that bad things can happen if you don't have your work all done.

Decades later, I still have perfectionist tendencies. I like things done right. I see that as a good quality, but it has its drawbacks. I have spent most of my married life trying to be on top of things despite ill health. To this day, when my family ask if they can help, my body tenses. Not all the time, but more often than not, I reply, 'It's okay, I'm fine, thank you. Most of it is done now. I'm just doing bits and pieces.' But the words are no sooner out of my mouth than I feel uncomfortable and on edge. I can't deny the thought that's going around in my head, 'No one can do it the way I like it done.'

It took my grandchildren to show me how much it means to them when I allowed them to help me. They've shown me how much fun making scones, cupcakes, or a sponge cake together can be. I still remember my granddaughter's face as she carefully cracked an egg into a bowl for the first time. I see how intently the boys watch me as they take turns putting in some flour and margarine or mixing the ingredients together. Their delight was something I had never experienced or believed possible.

Nowadays, all the parents of my pupils say their children love coming to my house for piano lessons. I know that it is a warm, vibrant, cosy family home. The fridge in our kitchen is covered with photographs of our five daughters, their husbands and our grandchildren, as well as friends who have supported Tommy and me over the years. The back garden is a mini playground that both Tommy and I created for our grandchildren. My years of gardening created a beautiful, calm outdoor space. Tommy and I are at the centre of a loving family.

Today, mothering means being present to my five grown-up daughters and my grandchildren. I listen and allow them to speak without interruption before they finish their sentences and without rushing to give advice. I am there for them to feel heard, understood and loved.

Nothing matters more when it comes to health and wellbeing.

Chapter 21

CHANGES AND HABITS THAT HELPED

Gradually, my life and my sense of wellbeing began to change. With David's encouragement, in my late forties, I fulfilled a lifelong wish to paint, and joined an art class. In my first class, I stood at an easel, moving uneasily from one foot to the other as I stared blankly at an empty canvas. When the teacher approached me, I admitted, 'I don't know what to do. I can't even draw a straight line.' He smiled, picked out a picture in the calendar hanging on the wall behind me, pointed to the top left-hand corner and said, 'How about painting what you see in this corner? It's just a blue square. Don't look at the whole mountain. Focus only on one small area at a time.'

Four weeks later, I completed a simple painting. It was enough to keep me in that class. Over the years, I've had the satisfaction of seeing framed pictures of mine hanging at local exhibitions. Our B&B guests have even purchased some of my paintings.

Another day, I told David, 'I don't mind being alone. It's just people I have difficulty with.' He thought momentarily, smiled and said, 'A cross has two beams, one vertical and the other horizontal. The upright beam represents our relationship with ourselves, and the horizontal one represents our relationship with others.' Then he smiled and added, 'We need both.' Through the work with my psychologist, I was learning how to relate to others, to create connections.

I also joined a karate self-defence course. After each class, I felt great. As well as benefitting from the exercises, I began to feel more at ease with people.

In one session, David told me that sensitivity, rather than depression, was my problem. He gave me something he had written:

> How can I develop self-esteem? The answer is – you don't have to do anything especially worthy to create or deserve self-esteem; all you have to do is turn off that critical, harassing inner voice. Why? Because that critical inner voice is wrong! Your internal self-abuse springs from illogical, distorted thinking. Your sense of worthlessness is not based on truth; it is the abscess at the core of hopelessness and helplessness.
>
> So, for the time being, forget the 'negative' and 'unconscious historical tape' and focus on generating all the wonderful resources you have been blessed with. Enrich your life with your creative talents and continue sharing them with your family and friends – but don't 'rescue' or 'enable' them. Just love and share your gifts with others. Instead of looking for what's wrong and fixing it, think of ways to enrich your life and those around you.

Another day, he reassured me, 'When you first get yourself well, you'll be able to help other people.' Something in me shifted that day. A few months later, he suggested I write self-help articles for a local magazine.

Years ago, when I was in college in Cork and Tommy was up in Clifden, I would write reams and reams of letters to him.

When David first proposed it, the idea seemed preposterous. 'You wouldn't have to write more than five hundred words,' he reassured me.

That same evening, I sat down and wrote an article entitled 'If I Can Do It – So Can You'. I posted it to the magazine editor. To my delight, my article was published, and I was invited to become a regular contributor. I used the pen name *Rebecca* to protect my identity. Over a hundred articles were published until I stopped in the late 1990s.

Here's an excerpt from one of those articles:

Therapy has radically improved the quality of my life. However, 29 electroconvulsive treatments (ECT) and years of psychotropic drugs have left me with a damaged nervous system. I still find that hard to cope with.

When I woke up this morning, the pain in my temples had returned with a vengeance. Nothing in my body worked.

The negative sensations were dreadful. In desperation, I cried to God, 'Please, help.'

I struggled to get up even though I felt like a robot. Somehow, I made my way to the kitchen and prepared a cup of tea. Then, I sat on a chair, like so many times before, with my hands around the outside of the cup. I felt the gentle warmth, which always comforts and consoles me. Tommy, ever watchful, looked over at me and said, 'You're deep in thought.' I replied, 'No, I'm in terrible pain.' He responded, 'I want to feel the pain with you.'

I was so taken aback by his words that I shot back,

'No. It's bad enough one of us going through it, God, not two.' He smiled and said, 'Well then, just like people on strike, I'll go out in sympathy with you.' Something about the idea and how he said it made me laugh. I remained sitting and reflected on the gifts of compassion and empathy and what a difference they can make.

A few minutes later, I stepped outside to get fresh air and headed to the front of the house. The atmosphere all around was bliss. I wondered, 'Why didn't I do this earlier?' Who could believe yesterday was cold and wintry and today is like summer? Everything in nature seemed peaceful and serene. I strolled up and down the path, hoping to absorb what I can only describe as the healing atmosphere around me. I listened to the birds singing to their hearts' content and felt at one with nature. I wanted to remain there forever.

For years and years, I suffered constant screaming pain in my temples as a result of the ECT. Normal painkillers wouldn't make the slightest bit of difference.

To this day, the gift of meditation remains close to my heart and means everything to me. David was the first person to introduce me to it. At the end of each therapy session, he would do what he described as a deep relaxation/meditation exercise with me. Many times my temples were in excruciating pain, but at the same time I felt deeply relaxed.

He guided me with positive, affirming words, nothing more. He assured me that the deep peace I experienced was always there, and I could tap into it at any time. Those practices made an enormous difference to my health and wellbeing. To get help with the pain in my temples, David sent me to a pain clinic. When the doctor there suggested prescribing an antidepressant, I froze. It was out of the question for me. I never went back. Most of my adult life had been lived in a daze, mechanically going about my days because of the pain. Eventually, David suggested a homeopathist whose work he knew, and that eased the pain somewhat. Acupuncture also helped.

When I was about to leave his consulting room, David would shake my hand and hold my jacket for me as I put it on. Thanks to his good example, I do the same now with my piano students. Next, he would look at me with his smile and say, 'Leave all that garbage you've been carrying here with me. I've got a large incinerator I can put it into.' I always had a much better day afterwards. As I made my way down the stairs, I would feel light-footed, brighter and more connected to myself.

I think back to moments in my childhood when I occasionally had this feeling of connection with myself. At age 12, in secondary school in England, before we left to go to Ireland, we had swimming classes, and I remember for the first time ever, coming out of the water and feeling like a totally different person. The real me. It was a flash in the pan, but the memory of the moment stayed with me. I've often wished I could recapture that fleeting feeling from that day.

One day when I was seven, standing in the house, absolute mayhem going on around me, my mother and father were screaming at one another. Maybe one of them shouted 'What the hell are you doing there?' or something, but suddenly from out of nowhere came the thought, *I am a good person.* It flooded my whole being. With it came the realisation: it doesn't matter what's going on around me, it doesn't matter what others are saying to one another, I am a good person. Where that came from, I have no idea, some deep, hidden part of me coming up to rescue me.

I first heard of the Ten Commandments in primary school. Number four, 'Honour your father and your mother,' has haunted me ever since. I fervently believed that it obliged me to obey my parents no matter what. Like a timid mouse, I 'honoured' whatever they told me. Even as an adult, I placed them on a pedestal.

I'm the eldest of seven children. I've always viewed myself as inadequate. I don't remember playing with any of my brothers and sisters. I vividly recall being locked out of our home in London and confined to our small, neglected back garden for hours when I was four years old.

One day, to my absolute astonishment, I stumbled upon a tortoise who had made its way through a dividing hedge. I kept this discovery a secret, fearing that my parents would disapprove. That tortoise became my reason for living. I spent hours observing his slow movements and the way he retreated in and out of his shell. In his company, I felt at peace with myself. This was my only companion.

I've survived many traumas, but perhaps the most painful was the absence of any relationship with my birth family. Tommy was surprised that none of my family ever came to visit me in hospital. Not long after my mother's death, I unfortunately had a major falling out with my brother.

Years later, my late sister called to make peace over the whole affair. She said, 'I don't remember what that was all about. From now on, let's stay in touch.' I agreed. Sadly, things did not work out as well as we hoped and I did not keep up contact with them.

To my surprise, more recently, another sibling visited and startled me by appearing unexpectedly and banging on the window. Looking at him was like facing a younger version of my father. I felt numb. As we spoke, painful memories and sensations welled up inside me. My brother recalled his own memories, and I found it hard to hear how distressing they were. I did my best to remain calm and friendly. While I managed the encounter well, it drained me.

Afterwards, the resurgence of painful memories took its toll on my body. A profound sadness, like a solid block inside me, stopped me in my tracks. Tears struggled to escape. I tried to distract myself by resuming my chores and going into town to buy garden compost, but my mood didn't lift. The encounter with my brother after 30 years hit me hard. I was disappointed that it had taken so much out of me.

I tried to reassure myself, saying, 'Breda, keep growing. You've come through so much. You can come through this, too. All is well.'

Decades of unresolved trauma can't be glossed over as if it never happened, and certainly not at one random meeting. Some wounds never heal.

Today, I am fortunate to have a healthy, loving family of my own. I recognise that I'm more sensitive than most people and feel vulnerable a lot of the time. I've had to learn to steady myself in the face of emotional upheavals, which has involved revisiting some of the 'rules' and expectations I've held all my life and considered non-negotiable.

For example, I believed it was my responsibility as the eldest to reconcile with my siblings. I travelled to Limerick specifically for that reason, but my efforts proved a disaster and only made matters worse.

Today, I'm questioning some of the core beliefs I've tried to live by, particularly in relation to my family of origin.

How can one love those who inflicted pain that doesn't go away? How can I love my siblings when I've been estranged from them for decades? We don't know one another anymore, if we ever did.

Is that simply Catholic Church teaching, or does it have more to do with our common humanity? Is compassionate understanding for all affected the answer I've been looking for? We all do things we regret, myself included. How am I to 'honour my parents'?

What happens when it's just a one-sided affair? From what I know of myself, I'm willing to release the past, but what about my sibling, who I assume is still exceedingly angry with me? Is that something I must continue to live with, or can it be resolved through prayer and God's grace? Is there something I can do, or is it best to let sleeping dogs lie?

When I was writing this book, I shared the manuscript with a wise friend. I emailed him about some of the questions and concerns I had, and he replied:

> I've always believed we honour our parents most by becoming our 'true' selves. That's all we ever wish for our

children – that they are true to themselves and become who they uniquely are. Your book is a powerful acknowledgement of what your parents have meant in your life. You have honoured them by speaking your truth.

It's a great bonus if we can love and get along with our siblings. We all need to feel part of a tribe. By nurturing bonds with our siblings, we keep alive a support network for ourselves and for our collective children. But nowhere is it said we should allow them to abuse us.

There is a time to give and not to give, a time to stay within the boundaries of self-respect and take care of ourselves, and a time to go the extra mile on someone's behalf. Given the trauma you lived through, you've needed to put distance between yourself and your birth family to allow yourself to heal. You're only just getting there now. The mandate you have carried for years about what you 'should' feel towards your family of origin is one of the many mandates you're finally challenging – and choosing to discard.

What a tragedy that solid bonds with my original family are missing.

The strong bonds with Tommy's relatives are also a wonder to behold. I feel comforted and compensated, knowing I'm part of a loving and dynamic family.

I've asked myself a million times: Why can't I fix this? Why can't I solve it? How can I relate in a meaningful way when my siblings don't know me?

For years, I've never considered that the root of the problem could be greater than the family I grew up in. Could it be that unresolved hurt, woundedness, and an inexplicable inability to understand one another are but the symptoms of a deep ancestral wound? Is it possible that no one person can solve the dilemma of intergenerational trauma that has been passed down through the generations?

It breaks my heart. I like to get along with everyone, but I have limits, and I'm learning to respect them. Perhaps I've played my part by breaking the cycle within my own offspring.

Saying 'Yes' when I need to say 'No' is like an addiction that has always had a grip on me. I watch myself slipping into self-defeating patterns of behaviour. But I am learning to speak out on my own behalf rather than endlessly trying to please.

I was asked to play the organ to cover the music in church for the Easter Penitential Service in 2024. I didn't want to go. Bad experiences over the years had developed into a phobia. But after reasoning with myself, 'I'm here to serve', I caved in.

Throughout the service, I was anxious. Some of the words the priest used made me cringe. They felt deeply insulting to me as a human being. Despite my many faults and failings, I did not see myself as a 'slave to the evil within me'.

My tummy became more unsettled as troubled emotions tightened their grip on me. I wondered how the service appeared to be acceptable to everyone else, but not for me. But I feared saying anything about my uneasiness to the priest.

The next day, I saw what I was doing yet again in my life. I was choosing not to speak in my own voice for fear of losing the approval of others, selling out on myself in the hope I would not offend them.

Catching ourselves as we slide into familiar self-defeating behaviour patterns is the prerequisite of change. Awareness brings with it the opportunity to choose to respond differently. I could say nothing, or I could share my concerns with the priest. To say nothing made me complicit. If I voiced my concern, perhaps I could make a difference.

I wrote the following email to him:

Good afternoon, Father.

As you know, I love your sermons and have done so for years. Perhaps that's why I felt disappointed in church last night. It all felt different. Since I was a little girl, I've had many bad experiences with the Sacrament of Penance, and I genuinely feel on edge if anyone even mentions the word confession. I wouldn't have been in church last night, only that I was asked to play the organ.

I tried to relax after I had played the entrance hymn. During the examination of the conscience ritual, I was appalled when I heard, 'For being a slave to the evil within me – Lord have mercy.' With great respect, I found those words offensive to my humanity.

For me, they seemed to obliterate any sense of the goodness within me that can never be destroyed. While imprisoned in a straitjacket and drugged intravenously against my will in St Brigid's Mental Asylum, Ballinasloe, I encountered that goodness and will never deny it again. I was upset and aggrieved when I got home last night and asked Tommy, 'How could any priest say that?'

Right now, I'm asking myself, 'Where is God's love in such words?' I hope you don't mind me sharing my deep upset last night. Perhaps it's an opportunity to make a change.

Within minutes, the priest graciously replied:

> Hello, Breda. I'm so very sorry about the upset last night caused you. I agree that the language in that penance rite is not helpful and is indeed hurtful. It is not the language I'd use myself; on reflection, I should have chosen a different format. Thank you, Breda, for your honesty. I send you my warmest regards for a blessed and peace-filled Easter.

I was overjoyed. To my surprise, the priest called me seconds later to make sure I was okay. I couldn't believe it, and he told me he wouldn't use that version again. It was lovely to think I had made a difference. I replied, 'I'm delighted that I told you instead of suppressing everything as I've done for years.' He agreed. For the rest of the day, I was happy with myself. I had never felt like that before.

However, four days later, I saw the same priest heading in my direction when I was in the town centre. He was out walking and passed very close to me, but instinctively, I hid behind the petrol pump so he wouldn't see me.

I was embarrassed. I worried about what I had said to him. As I crouched low out of sight, all I could think was, *What must he think of me now?*

Confronting that priest had taken every bit of courage I had. I wasn't simply challenging the language of some penitential rite; I was speaking out against a lifetime of shame-based preaching in the Catholic Church and confronting every male in an authority position that I had ever feared. What was at stake was that he may disapprove of me for being critical and hold that against me, as others had done before him.

I can see why I was hiding behind the petrol pump. This was all very new for me. It takes time to adapt to behaving differently. Like a new pair of shoes, it requires wearing them repeatedly to become comfortable in them. I am proud to have faced him, but I'm also compassionate towards my worries afterwards.

I've always divided myself into likeable and unlikeable parts. What if they're all me? What if my blended, mended, and gifted selves each have a critical place in my life? They have each played a critical part in making me who I am. Together, they make up my identity.

I know now that I need to work at feeling good in myself. I have many interests that keep me sane. I love being creative – gardening, home decorating, cooking, baking, reading, writing, art. I particularly enjoy being in the company of my music students. They give me a lift more times than they realise. I also appreciate the social aspect of chatting with their parents afterwards.

My faith is important to me. It steadies me. I pray when I'm uneasy or uncertain of some important choice I have to make. It brings me home to myself. It helps me be patient and trust that when I am open, the answers do come.

The mantra 'We all need support' has become a cliché, as though it is easy to find. For most of my life, I struggled hard with that. I couldn't access support anywhere. I had no one I could turn to. I was painfully isolated.

Since Tommy and I met, he has always been there for me. His constant support through very difficult periods of my life has been life-giving. But I've also needed someone independent who understood at a deep level why I felt so bruised and unable to cope with life. I was fortunate to meet such a person in 1995, a gifted counselling psychologist. David was my lifeline for many years until he died.

In addition to psychotherapy, I have found particular writers to be very helpful. Fiona Brennan's book, *The Positive Habit* and her excellent online courses kept me going through Covid. I found Wayne W. Dyer's words: 'Know that everything will happen at just the right time, at just the right place, with just the right people' most reassuring.

I've always needed good friends and wise people to believe in me and encourage me to be myself. Their acceptance has allowed me to trust myself.

During August 2021, I heard Gerry Hussey being interviewed on Midwest radio. He had just published a book entitled *Awaken Your Power Within*, which I read and loved. I reached out to him and became a member of The Soul Space Community in September 2021, founded by Gerry and his wife Miriam.

I began to develop a new lifestyle. Exercise and a positive mindset were paramount. I have also learned the importance of healthy eating habits and a flexible daily mental and physical health regime. The first thing I do when I wake up every morning is to drink a glass of water because of its scientifically proven health benefits.

I start my day with a guided meditation and again before I sleep at night. I access these through my phone. I like the resources available within the Soul Space Community: Thought for the Day, Reflections, Meditations, and Meditative Moments. When I'm at my wits' end, I find the late Louise Hay's affirmations and talks extremely helpful for reconnecting me with a positive take on my life.

Meditation has helped me to become stronger in myself and less reliant on external aids. It has taught me to be gentler and made it easier to be with myself and to ask for support when I need it.

Whether I'm stressed or not, one of my favourite pastimes and exercises is a walk to the beach. The other day, I was sitting on a rock at the beach, smiling. I had just gone out for a walk. As I stood on the white sand and watched in awe as the strong waves rolled in and out, I wondered if there was a way to allow my feet to feel the impact of those waves with their healing power.

But I had no towel. I wanted to walk further, but not with sand stuck to my feet. As I turned to leave, thoughts of Miriam and Gerry and how they had both stressed the importance of finding fun things to do occupied my mind. So I turned back. I let go of my worries about the sand. Standing in the sand barefoot with the waves crashing around me created a glorious feeling that seeped into every bone in my body.

Miriam invited us to write a poem entitled 'Being Me'. I had never written a poem before but decided to try it.

Being Me

Where would I be without the God of my strength?
How would I cope?
I don't know.
Get up in the morning.
Face the day ahead.
So many challenges.
Things to do.
I work hard to achieve it all.
I try to be loving.
I try to be kind.
I try to be all I'm meant to be.
I struggle and strive for all that's ahead.
But what if I stopped?
Just stopped.
Stopped to be me.
To enjoy being me.
To hear the silent call and know I'm doing okay,
Being me.

Over the past two years, one of the greatest assets I have gained as a member of the Soul Space Community is the 7 a.m. Activation Sessions online on Tuesdays and Thursdays. Jason Quigley, a professional boxer from Donegal, guides us through six to eight rounds of 'throwing punches' as well as cardio and core work. No matter how intense the session is, he wants it all to be a bit of craic and fun.

He christened us 'The Mighty Ducks' and set up a WhatsApp group. We have all become very close. Once a month, instead of boxing, we chat to get to know one another better. The camaraderie and knowing that we have one another's backs puts us in great form and sets us up for the day.

Last Christmas, Jason bought each of us a Bali T-shirt with the Mighty Ducks logo printed on the back and front. Whenever I put it on, I connect with and relish the irreplaceable feeling of belonging.

Jason always begins and ends the class with a beautiful meditation and inspiring words that come straight from his heart. The last round ends with Jason encouraging us to throw punches with 'high knees, fast hands' as we sing, 'We will, we will rock you'. It's a great workout, and the fun we have is extraordinary.

His empowering slogan, a quote by Tim Ferriss (an American lifestyle guru), is our emblem: 'Win the morning, win the day.' It's incredible how much energy levels soar after doing Jason's sessions.

Last Saturday, on my 75th birthday, my eight-year-old granddaughter sang a beautiful action song in our kitchen that she had learned in school: 'It's me (you, us) who build community.' The broad smile on her face said it all. Surrounded by family, I was ecstatic as we all sang along. Her vibrancy and energy as she did the actions held me spellbound. Her words captured what Soul Space Community has meant to me in my recovery.

Apart from my 21st birthday, my birthday was never celebrated, and even in my late twenties, thirties and forties, I didn't want my birthdate acknowledged here at home either. Seeing how differently birthdays are celebrated nowadays, especially with my grandchildren, finally won me over. Everyone's birthday is a wonderful occasion.

On the eve of my 75th birthday, Tommy brought me to Rosleague Manor Hotel in Connemara for dinner. Little did I know what had been planned. I couldn't believe my eyes when we entered the high-roofed and elongated sun porch where the bar was located. Sitting around a table at the end were Maria, Marguerite, Karen, and Michelle, our eldest granddaughter. I bubbled up with joy. It was a wonderful surprise.

When we sat down, the manager came over and talked to us for ages. A discussion arose about how difficult it can be for children growing up when their parents are heavily involved in running a business to make ends meet and can't be as present for their offspring as they would wish. There could be other reasons, an illness, a duty to perform or other urgent matters.

His words meant a lot to me. I felt comforted and consoled. I wasn't the only mother in the world who couldn't always be there for her children to hear their stories and be present for them during their formative years. I wasn't a businesswoman, but I have regrets about not being able to be there for them as much as I wanted to be because of emotional struggles.

We had an excellent meal – the food was delicious. Then, out of the blue, Maria said with a glorious smile, 'Mum, that's beautiful what you and Dad are doing for Francis and Peter with the little headstones.'

A wise friend had suggested that Tommy and I erect two

beautiful headstones in our local graveyard to also honour the memories of Francis, the baby I lost because of a miscarriage, and Peter, who was stillborn. I had sent a message to our WhatsApp family group explaining the plan.

I beamed at the mention but was surprised when Karen said, 'I feel a blockage around that. I gave it a thumbs up, but …' She stopped there.

I had a hunch that if I said more about what happened around the two deaths it might be helpful. They listened intently and seemed touched by the story that unfolded. Their responses were very affirming. 'Mum, how did you survive all that? How did you come through it? You're amazing.'

We talked about how, 40 years ago, people didn't regard communication with children as important, especially when it came to explaining the impact of a major crisis on families. Maria pointed out that Karen was four when I was pregnant. 'You would have seen Mum's tummy getting bigger. You would have been looking forward to a new brother or sister and then nothing.' Together, we made sense of what happened. This was a very healing conversation for all of us.

The staff arrived at our table with a birthday cake and sang 'Happy Birthday'. Other guests joined in. I was in my element.

My family and grandchildren who do not live nearby travelled to join us the next day. My granddaughter Allie sang and danced her heart out, and I got to accompany Diarmuid and Finnán on the piano as they played a French folk song and 'Twinkle, Twinkle Little Star' on the violin. Then, we all headed to the beach for a walk. Maria rushed to write 'Happy Birthday' in the sand. Her children added, 'We will always love you, Nanny.'

I couldn't help thinking of our three boys who died as babies: Dermot, Francis and Peter.

Tommy gave me a beautiful present of two nights away in the Lodge, Ashford Castle, County Mayo. As an extra surprise, Marguerite and Breda Ann will also join us. I couldn't be happier.

Chapter 22

WHAT'S GOD GOT TO DO WITH IT?

Throughout my life, I've wondered about the Being we refer to as God and by many other names.

I first learned about Him as a youngster sitting at the back of a special class to prepare us for making our First Confession. I listened intently to a strong-minded teacher describe Him as a stern figure who insisted on obedience to a broad set of rules. God seemed more interested in pointing out what we should not do than showing us how to live our lives.

I took to heart every word the teacher said, especially her warning that to tell a lie in Confession was worse than a mortal sin. I became terrified of a God who was out to punish me for any false move I made.

That fear intensified during my First Confession. In my mind, I had lied. I remember telling myself, 'My soul is black. Jesus can't come to me.' I was seven years old.

That same year, my fear of an angry God was compounded by guilt over having stolen money from my mother's purse. I had taken it to buy sweets for other children. When I confided this 'sin' in Confession, the priest responded harshly. He told me I could not be forgiven until I returned the money. Being unable to fulfil this obligation, I lived in dread of being punished.

As a family, we adhered to the strict rules of the Catholic religion. Once a month, we were marched to the church for Confession, whether we wanted to go or not. Attendance at

Sunday Mass was obligatory, as was the fast from midnight before receiving Holy Communion.

As I grew into adolescence, attending church came to be a welcome relief from the unbearable stress I lived under at home. Then came my three years as an aspirant and a postulant; those nuns passed on the harshness they had experienced in their formation.

God remained a distant, punitive figure for me until I encountered a priest working in a youth club near Kylemore Abbey, where I worked in my twenties.

I attended the club every Friday night and was drawn to this man's different take on religion. His concern and commitment to the young people was genuine. We all had great fun. I visited him sometimes for a chat. I always felt better afterwards. He showed me that God was kind and not at all the ogre in the sky who had haunted my life. He was the priest I asked to marry us. Tommy liked him, also.

Life moved on, and I continued to observe what was expected of me as a Roman Catholic.

I followed the status quo because I feared being seen as different. Even as a married woman, I attended Sunday mass 'religiously' to avoid conflict with my family. I also had a deep need to belong within the community.

During the 1980s and 1990s, I became involved in the Charismatic Movement, which sponsored prayer meetings across Ireland that were infused with upbeat folk music. There was always some criticism of these meetings as they were perceived to be fundamentalist and disrespectful of the orthodox Church. But they radically changed my concept of God. For the first time, I experienced God as far more loving and compassionate than I had ever realised.

Gradually, I've come to reject images of God that filled me with fear and terror. Today, I embrace a spirituality that speaks to me of beauty, mystery and unconditional love. I believe in a God who wants only the best for me.

I enjoy playing the organ once a fortnight for Saturday evening Mass or when called upon for funerals or other events. I appreciate reassuring sermons that relate to my life on any given day. Sometimes, it seems more than a coincidence that I hear the precise words that powerfully speak to me. Whenever that happens, I leave the church with a spring in my step. I feel empowered and ready to take on whatever comes my way.

There are other moments when I feel connected to the Sacred. This seems to happen when I reach out in the silence of my heart as I would in an ordinary conversation with someone I love. I say whatever is on my mind. I believe I'm talking directly to the Good Lord in His unseen presence when I do that. It's also the same with Our Lady when I turn to her.

I've learned that the Sacred is everywhere. To this day, I find that deep sense of belonging when I walk and connect with nature; I see it in my grandchildren's eyes and smiles.

My faith and my psychological difficulties have been two interwoven aspects of my life. At times, they have worked together, but they struggled with each other for many years. It was difficult to maintain consistent faith in a loving God when I was falling apart inside and unable to experience relief. I felt so disempowered that I yearned to be saved by a force much greater than myself. I had to learn that mature faith doesn't allow one to skip over emotional issues that must be faced and resolved. Faith doesn't give a person shortcuts or quick fixes.

I believe in the Jesus of the Gospels. I frequently turn to Him in meditation or when my back is against the wall. I sometimes feel frustrated when I don't get any response. But given time, something happens to lift my spirits, and my heart opens.

I lost three of my children as babies – Dermot, Francis and Peter – but I still feel connected to them. Similarly, other people meant a lot to me when they were alive, and even though they have since died, I still talk to them and enlist their help. I feel strongly connected whenever I do.

I relate to God in the same way. I call from my heart. I listen to the whisperings of my soul. I recall being confined in a straitjacket in St Brigid's Hospital until that wondrous afternoon in 1973 when my dad defied medical authorities and rescued me. On top of other psychotropic drugs, I was given 'Sodium Amytal grs three orally at night and repeat.' 'Nembutal grs, 4 plus 50mgs Largactil, intramuscular.' Repeatedly, I was drugged intravenously against my will.

For almost 11 days and nights, I battled for my sanity as I drifted in and out of a type of sleep that defies description. Then, one afternoon, lying in the straitjacket with straps across my chest and iron rails on either side of the bed, I discovered a place inside me that could never be destroyed, no matter what others at the time were doing to me.

My faith has sometimes been magical, but I hope it's different now. I trust it when it gives me faith in myself to face challenges and difficulties. When it allows me to let go of the past and open myself to new experiences in the present.

Chapter 23

LETTING GO OF RESENTMENT

Forty years ago, I felt unbearably guilty because I was unable to forgive my dead parents for all I had lived through. I went to see our local priest, who assured me this was normal and there was no need to be upset. Forgiveness is a process. I couldn't rest, though. In church, I felt a hypocrite when it came to saying the words of the Our Father. The lines 'And forgive us our trespasses as we forgive those who trespass against us' got to me each time. Under my breath, I changed the words to, 'As I *try* to forgive …'

No one ever told me how long it takes to move from anger to forgiveness. In my case, this was partly because I never realised how angry I was. I never thought of myself as an angry person, and when someone suggested that 'suppressed anger' might be at the root of my repeated panic attacks, I let him know I wasn't impressed.

I wasn't only angry. I was hurt and sad and permanently on edge. My parents had betrayed my trust through their lack of love, neglect and complete unpredictability. I still feel sad for that needy, insecure child who grew up in a chaotic world and blamed herself for the rejection and violence she experienced.

My inner life was layered with different emotions. It was simplistic to say that my problems were all due to 'suppressed anger' and that forgiveness would set me free of them. My inner life was alive and layered with negative emotions. It had to be unpacked before I could understand their hold on me.

Until I could name and express the range of feelings I carried inside me for years, I couldn't begin to consider forgiving those involved. It was late in my life that I recognised and accepted the harm that unresolved anger and resentment were doing to my health and close relationships. Only then could I step back from them and consider letting them go.

I did not need to feel ashamed for being angry, furious, and resentful. But I had to be careful not to allow suppressed emotions to turn into bitterness, cynicism and hatred.

I was in my seventies before I realised that I needed to go deeper, feel my intense, deeply embedded anger, hurt and rage, and healthily express my blocked emotions. My responses at the time were valid. Acknowledging what happened is essential to understanding why things turned out the way they did.

Recently, I took specific steps to face what had made me angry throughout my life. I drew up a list and didn't stop until I got it all on paper. I was surprised to see 54 examples of what had made me furious. I had stifled my anger for decades for fear of even worse happening.

Continuing with the exercise, I picked out the most striking ones and wrote about the advantages and disadvantages of holding on to my anger. Here are two examples of my reflections:

Example 1

I resent that I felt unloved as a child. I never got to learn how to love because I had no role models. I find myself bitter and furious over that now because of the knock-on effects it had on my ability to be a loving mother to my children in their childhood and formative years.

Advantages	Disadvantages
1. I have someone to blame.	1. I might like to think that blaming others has an advantage, but I'm achieving nothing. I'm only hurting myself.
2. My anger is justified.	2. Anger, resentment, and rage multiply by the day when I don't find a way to release these emotions and let them go.
3. By holding on to my hard feelings towards my parents, it lets me off the hook. Inwardly, I can reassure myself it was all their fault, instead of taking responsibility for my own actions and behaviours whenever I failed my children.	4. My anger, resentment, and rage prevent me from being the person I'm meant to be.

Example 2

Holding on to my anger means I never let the person who hurt me off the hook.

Advantages	Disadvantages
1. These strong, unabating, painful emotions remind me that I was almost raped on my first date. I have every right to be angry.	1. The man my anger is directed towards is not the person being hurt. My relations with people I care about now are affected by the negative energy that my unresolved anger generates.
2. My outrage validates how wrong he was to assault me. It is my way of punishing him for what he did. My being angry with him means he can never forget what he did.	2. Holding on to my anger and resentment does nothing to settle the score. I'm the only one suffering. He has moved on and probably forgotten it ever happened.
3. My anger is the proof I need of how badly I was treated.	3. I recognise all too well how badly I was treated in the past. Holding on to my anger simply allows those who hurt me to control my future.

After completing several similar exercises on my beliefs about the value of holding on to rage and resentment, I realised that the only person I'm hurting when I hold on to anger and years of built-up resentment is myself. The more I tightened my grip around these painful emotions, the more I allowed the people who harmed me to control my life.

Forgiveness in no way condones bad things that were done to me. It frees me to look at the bigger picture and appreciate the frailty of the human condition.

Choosing to forgive makes me a survivor who has freed herself from the steadfast grip of anger, rage, fury, fear and resentment. I'm no longer living my life imprisoned in a cell of my own making, where destructive emotions have the upper hand.

Forgiving implies choosing not to be a victim and letting go of our natural tendency to believe other people are making us feel the way we feel. I've spent a lifetime blaming others for how I feel, but now I have the ultimate choice of how I want to show up on any given day.

Forgiving myself and others has not been easy for me.

My siblings never forgave me for abandoning them and escaping to a convent in my teens. I've never forgiven myself for not screaming my head off when my dad's best friend chased me around the room and assaulted me. When I've tried to forgive myself for being so gullible, I hit up against an impenetrable wall of resistance.

I went to Confession for years but never felt absolved for any of the sins I made up and rattled off. When I was an aspirant and postulant in the convent, weekly Confession was obligatory. I had no sense of God being warm, kind, loving and forgiving.

In contrast, when I opened up to my therapist about how ashamed I was, I left his consultation room walking on air, full of joy. I felt I had been forgiven. Why couldn't Confession be as liberating?

The God I believe in now is a loving God. When I feel loved, it helps me accept myself as I am now, with all my vulnerabilities and insecurities, and, in turn, to accept others as they are.

I think about that child I was and what she survived. I hold her gently in awareness. I put my right hand under my left arm near my heart, and the other hand crossed over and rested on the top of my right arm. I feel comforted and reassured. Our pain, when cradled in self-compassion, unfolds in a different way. I own what I've achieved despite adversity and trauma, and I let go of shame.

Despite some sympathy for both my parents, I've struggled all my life to resolve my anger towards them. I've been unable to forgive them even though there were times when I believed I had. Carrying resentment in one's body over the course of a lifetime takes its toll. Unable to resolve my rage against them, I turned on myself for not being stronger and challenging their cruel behaviour. My unpleasant emotions have pulled me into a painful self-centred mindset where I become absorbed into bitter ruminations and succumb to self-pity. I realised that I would never be free until I could forgive. Feeling angry towards myself and others only perpetuated the damage I experienced.

In his book *No Bad Parts*, Richard Schwartz discusses how we can befriend the parts of ourselves that we dislike. I identified my inability to forgive as a part of myself that I have difficulty accepting. I completed an exercise that Schwartz recommended for getting to know this part of myself better. This involved relaxing my body and noticing any thoughts, emotions, sensations, and impulses that came into my awareness.*

Next, I imagined a conversation between me and what I called my 'unforgiving self'.

I asked my unforgiving self what she was trying to teach me, why she maintained such a strong hold over me, and what role she believed she was playing in my life. Schwartz suggests that there is a reason why unhelpful, destructive parts of ourselves persist, no matter how hard we try to banish them.

My unforgiving self replied: 'I'm here to protect you, as strange as that may seem.' She continued, 'I know well how wronged you have been, and I'm here to make sure that never happens to you again. I am armour around you that no one can penetrate.'

I acknowledged her protective role in my life and asked her what it would take for her to allow me to forgive those who hurt me. She replied: 'I need to know you're safe.'

I like things to be perfect; at least, as perfect as possible. I like things done right. That personality characteristic has been in me since I was a young child when I was first tasked with cleaning the kitchen. I got into the tiniest corners, cleaned and polished until everything shone bright. My attention to detail got me into trouble because I ran out of time. But I enjoyed the challenge; it made me happy.

I set high standards and find it impossible to accept anything less. I want to love my husband and my family, but I fail miserably

---

* Schwartz, Richard C. *No Bad Parts: Healing Trauma and Restoring Wholeness with the Internal Family Systems Model.* Boulder, Colorado, Sounds True, 2021, pp.26–7.

at times, and I feel bitterly disappointed in myself. I dismiss the gentle inner reassurances that I'm a human being like everyone else, doing the best I can.

I need to accept that imperfections are part of the human condition, and that's okay. They don't have the last say because, with patience, I can work on my faults and failings and grow.

I can also get to know more about those aspects of myself – my anger, sadness, fear and physical pain – that make it hard for me to accept and love myself.

Angry thoughts cause ripples of stress to course through my body, which becomes lodged in my abdomen. If I were to give it a colour, that colour would be the black of nuggets of coal, tightly fused and ready to burst into flames at the slightest provocation. My anger can give way to sadness, which I feel with painful intensity; grief for what I lost through years of neglect and abuse. A lonely part of me finds release through tears as I mourn the person I might have been if given half a chance.

Fear consumes my whole body when I sense that the past keeps repeating in my life, and I will never be free. Persistent pain is my body's response to the burden of carrying so much hurt inside me for so long.

My hope is that I will continue to grow, and I see evidence of that dotted throughout my life. What has become clear to me is that my recovery won't be achieved through an act of will that 'overcomes' or 'beats' these aspects of myself into submission, but through an act of surrender that acknowledges and befriends them. Healing depends on understanding that the hurt I feel is a legacy of my past but that my past does not have to dictate how I choose to live in the present. Healing is also an achievement of the heart. It begins when I relax the clenched fist in my mind and open my heart to befriending unconditionally what I have resented in myself, until now.

There is a place inside all of us that is inherently good and can't be destroyed. I experienced this place inside myself when hospitalised against my will in a mental asylum, confined in a straitjacket for 11 days.

I want to live in a way that allows me to stay connected to my essential goodness. When I am in touch with what is deepest in me, I am at peace. I'm a human being. I will always have my faults and failings, but they are not the whole story.

There's a sadness, a sense of remorse, and deep regret inside me that I can't quite explain but which I can choose to hold in awareness with compassion. I am 76 years old. I can own my anger at my parents and my guilt for those times when my children felt the consequences of my neglectful childhood.

I imagined what I would say to my parents now if I could open my heart and forgive them. This is what I think I want to say:

Dear Mammy and Daddy,
    Without you, I wouldn't be alive, and my children and grandchildren would never have come into being. I owe you both a lot. You both endured unrelenting terrors, the trauma of war and poverty-stricken circumstances, with little, if any, support.
    Daddy, you drank a lot to cope, and your violent outbursts and the demands made an already unbearable

situation worse. Mammy, you found yourself a downtrodden wife and mother left alone to bring up seven young children. You had a husband with a severe alcohol problem who ruled the roost and rendered you powerless.

You were unable to bond with me due to unresolved generational trauma. We both suffered the loss of a close relationship that might have brought joy into our lives. I, in turn, found it difficult to mother my own children.

Sometimes my anger bubbles to the surface. I've realised lately that I hold on to rage and resentment so that I won't ever forget how badly I was treated. Part of me wants to scream from the rooftops, 'I was right, you were wrong.'

How do I let go of my anger and rage? As I see it, I have two choices. I can continue to live my life within the narrow constricts of victimhood, or I can let go my desire for revenge. I've carried resentment for most of my life, and I'm now in my 70s. My negative thoughts and emotions affect my entire body and make it hard for me to feel good about being alive.

Who am I fooling? I need to release emotions that no longer serve me. I need to forgive you both. This is my choice, my decision. It's up to me. Today, Mammy and Daddy, I no longer wish to harbour angry, resentful feelings. I forgive you both, I wish you well.

Breda

I have regrets about my own behaviour also. I feel ashamed for what I put my body through. I may never have been aware of what I was doing in asking it to carry so much unresolved pain, but I am powerfully aware now. To my body, in a frank and heartfelt way, I want to say I'm sorry.

I want to say these words from my heart, not my anxious mind. My inability to forgive kept me stuck in a quagmire of agonising, torturous thought patterns for years.

I grieve for the stress and suffering I brought into Tommy's life. What I put him through when I attempted suicide is something I couldn't bear to think about until very recently. For long stretches of our marriage, I was more of a burden than a companion. But maybe I've carried that weight of regret for long enough.

Forgiveness is one of the hardest things for human beings, but it is also one of the greatest gifts we can give ourselves. After a massive struggle to get there, it's a choice for me.

I can stay stuck in unforgiveness and continue to beat myself up, or I can choose to be hostage to my rage and regret no longer. Today, it's time to let it go. To enjoy a new freedom within by releasing a lifetime of unresolved guilt, anger and remorse.

I choose to set this bird free of its cage and make something beautiful out of the shrapnel of my past.

Chapter 24

ACCESSING MY MEDICAL FILES

One of the important steps I took in my recovery was finding out exactly how I had been diagnosed in psychiatric hospitals, the medications I was prescribed, and what precisely was going on when I had to undergo 29 ECT treatments.

This information was contained in my medical files in five psychiatric hospitals where I had been admitted between 1972 and 1990. Accessing these records, with their notes and reports and letters of discharge, could provide a different perspective on my condition and verify and flesh out my memories of what happened. But the entire process proved to be harder than I had anticipated.

In 2001, I wrote to various psychiatric institutions and requested a copy of my medical records through the Freedom of Information Act (FOI). St John of God Hospital, Stillorgan, Dublin, told me they were a private hospital and did not come under the FOI Act. Under no circumstances could my records be released.

Sixteen years later, on 24 May 2018, the GDPR was signed into law. Finally, I gained access to my medical files from St John of God Hospital and my GP records.

When I first contacted St Patrick's Hospital, Dublin, in 2001, they also informed me that they didn't fall under the FOI Act, but if I attended in person, I could view my file.

Tommy and I visited the hospital in 2001, having arranged to meet with a psychiatrist who would show me my file. We were escorted down to a large room and invited to sit at the table in the middle of the floor while we waited for the designated doctor to arrive. I felt on edge as I paced the room and looked out at familiar buildings. I was determined that no one would get the better of me this time. Never again would I be detained in a mental hospital.

A psychiatrist I had never met joined us and sat across the table from Tommy and me. He opened my file, and a long silence followed. I asked politely, 'Please, can I see my medical reports?' He replied, 'I'm sorry, they're only open for discussion.' His response jolted me. I responded, 'But I was told over the phone that I could see them for myself if I came to the hospital.' He replied, 'I'm sorry. I can't let you view them. It's hospital policy.'

I needed to know what had happened from a medical point of view after I was first admitted in 1972. I said, 'I'd like to know what the reports say about my first few days in the hospital. I asked to go home but wasn't allowed even though I was a voluntary patient.' He flicked through the file and informed me that my behaviour at the time was viewed as 'hyper-manic'.

He seemed hesitant about giving me more information. He tried to discourage me from following my quest and told me it was common practice at the time for medical files to be updated every three or four days, and that was why there were numerous frustrating gaps in my file.

However, much to my surprise, in April 2022, when I was allowed access to my entire file online through the GDPR Act,

I discovered a substantial amount of information, nurses' notes with daily entries and other essential facts that were helpful to me. A harm test result was required before my records were released under GDPR. A black marker was used to blot out information here and there. I found a copy of some missing pages in other hospital files.

However, he explained to me that my treating psychiatrist at the time had withdrawn my hospital reports to have them available in his office when I went for appointments. He assured me that it wouldn't happen today without copies being put in place. When the psychiatrist died three years later, his wife was permitted to burn any patient records she came across in her husband's filing cabinet. Unfortunately, mine were included in that bundle.

I mentioned that our family doctor in Limerick insisted that I should never have been given ECT treatments and that I was 'treated wrongly' in both St Brigid's Hospital and St Patrick's Hospital.

I expressed my concern that patients are still being treated with ECT today. He tried to persuade me that the administration of ECT was down to a fine art. 'Extreme care is taken with each procedure, and every detail is monitored and accurate. The patients under my care receiving ECT treatments are over 60 and have benefited.' I listened and said nothing.

I wanted to challenge him and ask, 'What about the traumatic impact on the human body and the long-term damage that I, for one, have to live with for the rest of my life?' But I remained silent.

As our meeting came to a close, I commented, 'Before I go,

I'd like to say it's a pity we weren't able to get together sooner. Doing so would have saved us a lot of frustration and time.'

He replied, 'When a patient looks for their medical records through the Freedom of Information Act rather than going directly to the hospital, a certain protocol must be followed.' We shook hands, thanked him, and departed.

I was disappointed that I didn't get to read the file myself. For the next few months, whenever I came across a newspaper article that included scientific evidence about the dangers of ECT treatments, I posted a copy to the psychiatrist. He acknowledged my letters but never once commented on the research findings.

On 3 June 2020, John Read of the University of East London said there is 'no place' for ECT in evidence-based medicine due to the risks of brain damage. My experience supports these findings.

Read, a professor of clinical psychology and the study's lead author, describes previous research justifying the use of ECT in the UK and around the world as 'the lowest quality of any I have seen in my 40-year career'. The paper concedes that 'the severity and significance of the brain damage and memory loss (following ECT) is rarely studied'. It suggests that the placebo effect may explain why some patients find ECT helpful.* The research published in the *Ethical Human Psychology and Psychiatry* journal concludes, 'The high risk of permanent memory loss and the small mortality risk means that its use should be immediately suspended.' I couldn't agree more.

---

* Easton, Mark. 'ECT Depression Therapy Should Be Suspended, Study Suggests.' BBC News, 3 June 2020, www.bbc.com/news/uk-52900074.

My academic memory, including four years of university studies, has never returned, nor has my ability to play the classical pieces I had learned since my teenage years right up to my Bachelor of Music degree. As I am now 76, I would classify that as permanent memory loss.

In 2001, when through the FOI Act, I requested my medical records from the psychiatric unit, Galway, a photocopy of my file was sent by registered post. Reading through this for the first time hit me hard. I worried that my children would read those notes and see their mother in a negative way. I worried how this would make them feel about themselves. Could they also experience the mental anguish their mother endured? To save them from this level of confusion and self-doubt I decided it was best to destroy that early file.

In March 2022, for the purposes of this book, under GDPR I went in search of my records from St Pat's, St John of God Hospital and my GP reports. These files remain intact.

Unfortunately, when I tried to get a second copy of my file, despite the best efforts of GDPR, my medical records from the Psychiatric Unit in Galway were not found.

Health Service Executive

15 July 2022

Dear Ms O Toole,

I refer to your request, received in this office on 10 June 2022, made under Data Protection Legislation, for access to records held by the Health Service Executive (HSE).

In your request, you are seeking access to copies of

your medical records, which may be held by the Psychiatric Unit in Galway University Hospital since 9 February 1976 and earlier. Despite an exhaustive search under the names of Breda O Toole and formerly Breda McMeel, it has not been possible to supply copies of the aforementioned records. Thorough searches were conducted in respect to both names.

If you are unhappy with this decision, you may make a complaint in writing to the Office of the Data Protection Commission, Canal House, Station Road, Portarlington, County Laois. This will involve an independent investigation of the matter by the Data Protection Commission.

Yours sincerely,

Data Protection Decision Maker.

However, I had sufficient information from other hospitals and GP records about my admissions to the Psychiatric Unit in Galway, so I didn't pursue the matter.

Overall, I learned some key facts about my relationship with psychiatric services over 23 years:

1. I was admitted once to St Patrick's Hospital for four months.
2. I was admitted to St John of God for a couple of months on one occasion and for two weeks on another.
3. I was admitted to St Brigid's, Ballinasloe as an inpatient on three occasions. I also attended as an outpatient for ECT treatments.
4. I was referred to St Joseph's Hospital in Limerick, but the

medical director decided it was no fit place for me to be seen and sent me to Milford House instead for two weeks.

5. I was admitted to St Vincent's psychiatric unit, Elm Park Dublin, on one occasion.
6. I was admitted several times to the psychiatric unit in Galway.
7. I was held in a straitjacket for 11 days in St Brigid's Hospital, Ballinasloe.
8. As a patient in five Irish mental institutions, psychiatrists misdiagnosed, labelled, and treated me for severe illnesses that included bipolar disorder, Parkinson's disease, epilepsy, alcoholism, borderline personality disorder and hysterical personality.
9. From 1972 to 1995, I was prescribed multiple psychotropic drugs that produced very unpleasant side effects in my body. For ten years, I was seriously addicted to Valium tranquillisers.
10. I received ECT on 29 occasions, which has left me with chronic pain in both my temples and throbbing sensations in my head. Even with sheet music in front of me, I have also lost all memory of all of the classical piano pieces I ever learned, even in university.

When I began to read these reports and notes in 2022, I was surprised by the emotional upheaval they provoked. I felt a pervasive sense of upset as I revisited memories of sad and distressing times. I had a wide range of reactions, from grief to rage. There were times when I cried in frustration as my tummy pulsed with pain. I felt a huge range of emotions as I read them.

In my medical notes and formal letters between doctors

and services, I encountered a young woman who was hard to reconcile with who I am today. My heart went out to her for the pain she was in and the very superficial, dismissive way in which she was treated.

I was shaken by seeing my father's signature as the person who consented to me being administered ECT. He did so without any discussion with me. I was in my early twenties.

It was hard to read what others thought of me from a professional point of view when I was vulnerable. Reading the nurses' reports felt like being back in hospital again. I was disappointed by how distressing I found it to revisit my memories of them. I believed I had come to terms with those experiences way more than I actually had.

My feelings made sense when I confided in a friend about my reactions, and he wrote back to me, 'We can't erase or forget what happened to us; we can only befriend it. We face, feel, and express our pain and gradually make it part of the evolving story of who we are. We don't forget distressing experiences; we grow in our capacity to hold them.'

I needed to befriend the feelings that reading these records provoked rather than push them away. That didn't mean condoning bad experiences or minimising their impact.

First, I had to recognise and accept them without feeling diminished as a person. Writing the facts was one thing, but I was surprised by how difficult it was for me to acknowledge my feelings, face them and feel them.

As I confided to our local priest, 'It's as if the past has become alive in the present.' There were times when I felt my head was going to explode. He felt I needed more support to help me go through this process and recommended a psychotherapist he trusted.

I attended her fortnightly for 18 months. I read the draft chapters I was writing which I found particularly upsetting and discussed what they brought up in me. I felt safe doing so, and she was a profoundly compassionate listener. She kept me sane.

One thing I discovered was that I could easily slip into a mindset where I blamed life, my parents, the Church and psychiatry for ruining my life and lapse into self-pity. All that achieved was to reinforce my feelings of powerlessness and helplessness. I needed to stop seeing myself as a victim.

I took a course with Dr Edith Eger, whose book *The Choice* details the traumas she endured in Auschwitz in the aftermath of the Second World War. One of her mantras is no matter what horrors and abuses life has visited on us, we further disempower ourselves by assuming the identity of 'victim':

> We are all likely to be victimised in some way in the course of our lives ... This is life. And this is victimisation. It comes from the outside. In contrast, victimhood comes from the inside. No one can make you a victim but you. We become victims not because of what happens to us but when we choose to hold on to our victimisation. We develop a victim's mind – a way of thinking and being that is rigid, blaming, pessimistic, stuck in the past, unforgiving ...

I experienced darkness, pain, sorrow, joy, and good times. Each played an important part in shaping the person I've become. My difficulties and tragedies revealed an inner strength

I never realised I had. My lifelong struggle to find inner peace shows me who and what matters to me most in my life and what particular injustices I want to challenge.

Accessing my medical records revealed how lost and worthless I felt. They also showed me a person who survived and remained determined to understand why she felt so bad. Sadly, my records confirmed how, over 23 years, no one had taken the time to get to know me as a person and treat me with dignity. The consultant psychiatrist's female colleague at St Vincent's psychiatric hospital who showed me care and respect was a rare exception. Her conclusion at the time was that in spite of how distressed I was, there was no evidence that I had a 'mental illness'.

It concerns me that even when there is clear evidence of misdiagnosis in a patient's case, no protocol or law exists that requires a service to rectify the misinformation and remove erroneous and potentially damaging labels that continue to be attached to a person.

Reading the notes, assessments and reports written about me, I have formed a more complete picture of what happened to me. I can see why my problems seemed to worsen following hospital admissions and why my inner world became increasingly frightening and confusing for me.

Chapter 25

WRITING THIS BOOK

English was my downfall in school. I couldn't wait for the class to be over.

Writing an essay was terrifying. I tried hard to use my imagination, only to discover I had none. The words I wrote seemed random. In my mind, I was clearly the worst in the class. Somehow, I passed the Irish State examinations, but only barely.

Many years later I sought counselling to help me come to terms with experiences that had affected my health. In therapy sessions, I struggled to find the words to describe how I felt. I began to write down ahead of time what I wanted the therapist to know. To my surprise, I found solace in writing. It has remained my preferred way of communicating thoughts and feelings.

One day, my therapist suggested that I compile a series of articles from my journals and submit them to a magazine. To my surprise, my articles resonated with readers, and over a hundred were published.

My therapist subsequently encouraged me to write a book. 'You could include your published articles,' he said. I spent two years writing a book titled *Journey Towards Recovery – If I Can Do It, So Can You*. However, the disappointment of being rejected by several publishers led me to abandon the idea and refocus on my music career.

Some years later, I was captivated by a radio programme in

which a man described his outrage at being given electroconvulsive therapy at age 16. The presenter, Tommy Marren, invited listeners with similar experiences to call into the programme. I picked up the phone and was invited to do a radio interview. There were strong reactions to my contribution and calls for me to write a book, but I couldn't bear the thought of another rejection.

In 2021, I listened with interest to a talk by Dr Tony Bates entitled 'Begin Again'. His challenge to mental health services to ask, 'What happened to you?' rather than 'What's wrong with you?' struck a chord with me. I emailed him and attached an account of what had happened to me in St Brigid's Hospital, where I had been left in a straitjacket for 11 days before my father defied medical staff and rescued me. In a warm-hearted reply, he said, 'You have an important story to tell, and you're a gifted storyteller. I would be honoured to help you in any way I can to complete it and get it published.' I decided to give writing another chance.

I began drafting chapters that became this book. In my mind, I was writing to help people like me who had been hurt and confused by their experiences in psychiatric care. However, from Tony's perspective, my writing was primarily to further my own healing. 'If others are helped, that's a bonus,' he said. Hearing this, I protested, 'But I am healed.' Looking back, I smile now at my naivete.

At that time, I was experiencing spasms of pain that coursed through my body on a daily basis. I also suffered from blinding headaches, which had been a problem for years. I never mentioned these to anyone. I was terrified of being labelled 'mentally ill' again.

Through writing about events in my life I had tried hard to

forget, I was forced to re-experience them, as though for the first time. I recognised that I was not nearly as 'healed' as I wanted to believe I was. Writing this book over the past four years has been an important part of my recovery. It has required me to revisit difficult experiences, recognise their impact on my life and my relationships, and discover a gentler, more compassionate way of managing my vulnerabilities.

I couldn't have done this alone. Coming to terms with these and other traumatic experiences has taken time, support from mentors, and understanding, kindness and compassion for myself.

It has been a slow process. I have been supported by people who listened and 'got' my pain. They believed in me when I had no faith in myself. They allowed me to be myself, with my faults and foibles, and speak my mind without fear of judgement or rejection. My own family have also encouraged and supported me to tell this story, even if that meant re-opening and facing old wounds.

A friend recently wrote to me and described the path to personal healing as a 'Call to Adventure':

> When we hear this call to adventure, we often refuse the call and try to stay exactly how we are. From reading the stories of old, this seems to be an intrinsic part of every hero's journey. We say no as often as we say yes to the call to adventure. But the call is something we can never completely silence. It's that small voice in the quiet of our hearts that invites us to do something more with our lives. What it promises in return for our 'yes' is a path in life where we can

discover and embody our own truth and speak with our own voice.

Where that path leads us is entirely unknown and unpredictable. We may get hurt because every hero is wounded in some way; we may even die or experience a profound letting go of some part of our familiar selves that feels like a profound loss. In every heroic quest, someone or something dies; the journey may be a messy affair that inevitably takes us through places of confusion and darkness.

We need to be attentive and open to the supports that life offers us along the way. The heroes of all time have been graced with 'spirit guides' to show them their way.

These guides may be our teachers, our therapists, through whom we learn key skills to survive and complete our journey. They can be firm with us and expose our tendencies to read things in the wrong way and bring about our own downfall. They show us how tiny adjustments in our navigation can bring us through troubled waters, and they show how we may need to accept what is broken and hold it with compassion, viewing it not as some obstacle but as something that gives us a unique way of seeing in the dark.

I am indebted to wise guides I have been able to access in different ways, some via media platforms, for the wisdom and encouragement they shared from their own hero journeys:

Eckhart Tolle, Dr Gabor Maté, Fiona Brennan, Gerry and Miriam Hussey, Rumi, Thich Nhat Hanh, Louise Hay, and others. Their words often lifted me and reignited hope when I lost my way.

By facing and coming to terms with my past, I'm more open to taking risks in the present. One of my most recent journal entries reads: 'Not in my wildest dreams would I have ever thought I'd have the courage to do what I did yesterday when for most of my life the only way I could cope with animals and even birds was at a distance.'

Given the opportunity to participate in an activity at the School of Falconry, I overcame a deep-seated fear of animals and allowed a hawk to land on my arm. To my surprise, this was something I wanted to do.

First, I was introduced to a hawk, named Swift after the writer Jonathan Swift. The instructor gave an exciting talk about his daily work with the birds. Respect for their freedom is vital.

Next, we headed off into the woods. Swift followed us overhead, flying from tree to tree before swooping down to land on my gloved fist. This continued for over an hour.

I was delighted with myself. Whenever Swift landed on my arm, I connected with a place in my heart where I believed in myself. I stepped into the moment, established eye contact and connected with her. It was thrilling.

After Swift had eaten food off the glove on my right arm, I assumed she'd fly away. But she remained on my arm without any sign of moving. I was delighted she felt safe with me. The instructor said, 'She'll leave when she's ready.' And that's exactly what happened.

WRITING THIS BOOK

Swift taught me not to care so much about what other people think. She does her own thing when she's ready, and that's it.

But within a day or two of returning home, I was exhausted. Going to bed for a while helped, but my body still hurt when I got up again. The trip had been wonderful but had taken a lot out of me, partly because I had pushed myself too hard to reassure everyone I was having a great time.

I get frustrated by my persistent vulnerabilities and insecurities. I worry that trauma will remain the defining feature of my life and that recurrent jolts from the past will drown out the joys of the present.

Knowing that they pass helps me stay grounded during times of uncertainty and distress. I don't take things so personally anymore. I don't interpret my struggles as 'my fault' or as evidence of some personality deficit. Everyone has their ups and downs, challenges and exciting times. Why should my life be any different?

While some people find positive affirmations silly, I find them very helpful. I use them to nurture a more optimistic outlook and prevent my mind from being hijacked by thoughts that drag me down.

I no longer buy into the illusion that life is fantastic for everyone except me. I'm not alone in having off days. The more I talk to people, the more I appreciate that life is unpredictable, and we are all vulnerable. I'm not unique in finding myself from time to time in a difficult place.

What made my emotional struggles confusing was people writing off my distress as some form of 'mental illness'. Whereas there was always a good reason why I felt and behaved as I did, professionals rarely took the time to get to the root of my pain and help me deal with real issues in my life. They attributed my pain exclusively to some underlying brain disease or chemical imbalance. With each new psychiatric diagnosis I received, I felt less and less empowered. I became increasingly frightened of my inner world, which was governed by forces beyond my control. The best I could do was to avoid my feelings by staying busy. I was deeply ashamed of vulnerabilities and hid them as best I could.

A friend recently wrote to me during a tough week. His words rang true to me:

> Work has always been how you pushed through trauma. It strikes me that you put a lot of energy into proving to people you're not mad. Have you ever considered doing precisely the opposite? There is some madness in all of us, and you're no different. We live in a very unpredictable and broken world. No matter what we may say, we are all vulnerable. Sometimes, we worry and fear the worst; we overreact to bad news and momentarily lose our minds when old wounds are triggered.
>
> Sanity is not about becoming immune to any of the above. Mental health is about recognising the full spectrum of our raw and sensitive inner lives and befriending hurt parts of ourselves that the world didn't recognise, welcome or support.
>
> Your emotions can feel all over the place at times. The more we appreciate what you've survived, the less surprising that is. All you ever wanted was to be your-

self. But you grew up in a terrifying world where that was never encouraged. Where love was missing, you built protective defences to survive. And you live with an underlying dread that those defences will be breached.

What's impressive is that you've achieved so much, that you survived and enjoy life as you do. You held on through incredibly tough times and gave the world some of its most beautiful citizens.

Your pain has carved a deep empathy in your soul and care for many people whose lives have also been complicated.

But that doesn't mean your vulnerabilities have been erased. We grow not by 'overcoming' or 'exorcising' our demons but by befriending them, making room for them and putting out a welcome mat for them.

Your 'madness' has made you human. Stop apologising for it. I should get you a T-shirt that reads, 'I may be mad, but I'm also human.' On the back, we can write, 'And you should see what I've survived!'

Last night, I had a dream. A middle-aged woman, a stranger, was speaking to a crowd around her. In a clear voice, she said, 'It's madness to be living your life concerned about what other people think. It's madness to be living in fear of what might never happen. It's madness not to listen to your instincts and trust them.'

I enjoy life now more than ever before and live it fully. I remain as vulnerable as I've ever been. There are days when my heart aches, and my body hurts intensely. Recovery has made me more rather than less sensitive. Life gets to all of us when we open our hearts rather than keep it at a safe distance.

The gift of recovery is that I welcome new opportunities to grow and experience being alive more fully. Having convinced myself that other people had dreams and goals but not me, I can now see clearly how much I have to live for, and I'm determined to savour every moment I have left.

Chapter 26

A PLACE OF BELONGING

On Sunday, 30 July 2023, our golden wedding anniversary, like most mornings, I woke at 6.30 feeling stuck to the bed, with my body barely functioning and energy levels so low that getting up seemed impossible. Momentarily, I was angry that, similar to my wedding day, little in that line had changed. I was still prone to the residue of tense, anxious dreams and nightmares about being a patient in a mental institution. I wondered if doing a guided meditation would help but decided to get up instead.

I couldn't believe my eyes when I saw white wedding anniversary balloons in the piano room where I teach and in the kitchen, which also had a beautiful banner across the window that read 'Happy 50th Anniversary'. The number 50, dangling below, caught my attention. I stood motionless in time, felt the tears coming, and let them out while at the same time thinking, *This isn't how it's meant to be. Who cries on such an occasion?* I had mixed emotions. The way my daughters had so beautifully decorated the place for the occasion when I was asleep the night before filled me with enormous joy and delight. But my body was in pain and that wasn't easy to bear.

No one else was up, and I found comfort in being free to be myself and cry if I wanted to. The tears flowed. Fifty years! As never before, I saw all I had lived through, and again today, I was struggling.

I relaxed over a cup of tea and a slice of toast. Then, I felt a strong urge to go for a walk. I wanted nothing more than to be out in nature to feel connected to something above my everyday experience. As I walked down the road in the rain, I longed to experience a strong connection, a heartfelt bond with our three sons, who had died as babies. I spoke out their names, 'Dermot, Francis, Peter'. I wondered if the raindrops were tears from heaven of those who have passed on reaching out to me with love, compassion and empathy. Again, I sobbed my heart out.

When I arrived at the beach, I walked down the steps of the steep embankment, turned left, and made my way across the sand. By the time I had reached the far end, all I wanted to do was gaze at the vast expanse of the ocean. Standing motionless, I felt a strong sense of peace, strength and courage.

Just as I was about to leave the beach to walk around another one nearby, once again, all I could think of was the 50 years I had lived through. Life has its ups and downs, but to my mind, I had been through more than my fair share. As I climbed the last concrete step up onto the road, it occurred to me that not physically but emotionally, I still had open wounds from all the pain, hurt and trauma. The rain continued to lash down, but I had wet gear on, so I was okay. I stepped onto the pier wall and prayed amidst the vast sky and ocean.

After a few minutes, I left that spot and began to walk home. I noticed two neighbours in high-vis vests with another gentleman, a close and dear family friend, standing near his tractor. As I approached, I said, 'This is like a village gathering.' We laughed. I felt safe and happy. A few minutes later, I moved on but instinctively looked back and said, 'Tommy and I are 50 years married today.' They were all surprised and replied, 'Congratulations.' One said, 'Lucky man.' I replied, 'It's the other way around.' We burst out laughing, and instantly, my mood lifted. I was living life in a happier space.

By the time I arrived home, I was drenched but happy. I took off my rain-soaked clothes and wandered into the kitchen. Fiona, our eldest daughter, was there sitting on the armchair. The exact minute I entered the room, Tommy came through the other door. The timing was perfect. An image came to my mind: Tommy and I walking towards one another as if we were meant to meet. I will never forget that moment. For me, there was something out of the ordinary about the coincidence that was sublime.

Then it was congratulations from our family and a delightful time together opening presents. Tommy handed me a gift of gold Tree of Life earrings. The symbolism represents energy, health and a lovely future and alludes to the interconnection of life on this planet.

For the next hour or two, I sat peacefully and relaxed in the armchair, captivated by the scene unfolding around me. The kitchen was crowded with our 12 grandchildren and their mums and dads. I recalled the days when Tommy and I started as two individuals and nobody else in the kitchen existed. That was a wondrous moment. Without the two of us, everyone else, the mums, the dads and our grandchildren wouldn't be here.

I appreciate that taking quiet moments is essential, even on happy days. So I slipped into bed and listened to a short reflection on stepping into the here and now. Then, I decided to write about the day so far.

There was a quiet knock on the door, and Marguerite asked me if I'd like to come to town for coffee. 'Dad said he'll come if you do too.' I jumped at the opportunity to be with family again in a different setting – an experience I would never get again. The rain was bucketing down, but that didn't interfere with our enjoyment of the day. I found that realisation excellent, one to observe and savour.

Late that evening, Tommy and I, alongside our eldest granddaughter Michelle, headed into town as Fiona, our eldest daughter, wanted to give her electric car a top-up charge. On the way, she mentioned we would meet up with the others at the church car park to arrive at the hotel simultaneously. I saw nothing unusual about that.

So, after the car was charged, we pulled in at the church. Fiona and Michelle jumped out and said, 'Let's go and light a couple of candles.' I was a bit taken aback, but considering the day in it, why not? It would be nice to mark things that way, too, but I couldn't help laughing and said to them both, 'Gosh, you've become more religious than me.'

The entrance hall into the church was somewhat dark as it would usually be at that time of the evening. But when I turned right to go into the main body of the church, I was startled. The whole place was lit up; all the lights had been turned on, and the surroundings were much brighter than I had ever noticed.

The priest I greatly admire was the first to catch my attention. He was standing in front of the altar, and my eyes boggled when I saw all the adults of our family sitting in the front pews. I hadn't a clue what was going on. Then, Breda Ann handed me a bouquet, and that's when I knew for the first time that Tommy and I were about to walk up the aisle as if it was our wedding day. Not sure what to do, I held back until I heard Breda Ann say, 'Go on, Mammy.'

I was in fits laughing, and around the church, everyone seemed to be caught up in the laughter; the atmosphere was out of this world. The priest didn't know that Tommy and I hadn't an idea what was happening; it was all great fun. What followed was the most beautiful experience I could ever have hoped for. As we passed, some began singing, 'We're going to the chapel, and we're going to get married …' I laughed. When we eventually reached the top, the priest gave us time to sit, relax and enjoy the moment. I was still laughing. I think we all were because I could hear others laughing behind me. Then, the priest invited Tommy and me up to the front of the altar. After congratulating us, he read a short passage from St Paul, 'Love is patient, love is kind …'

Then he said he would bless our rings. Tommy replied, 'Mine won't come off.' There was an outburst of laughter around the church, me included. I got an idea and put my hand on Tommy's so that both our rings could be seen. These were intimate moments. I felt a strong, deep sense of connection. We renewed our marriage vows, and the priest read a beautiful marriage blessing by the late John O'Donoghue. I loved the sentiments expressed, especially the last line: 'As twilight harvests all the day's colour – May love bring you home to each other.'

The priest said:

> This is a fantastic moment. We ask God's blessing with great gratitude for life, love, and all you are about to

celebrate. I love weddings; most people do. It is a beautiful celebration of wishing couples well. But there's nothing at all that compares with this. Fifty years of living out through thick and thin is different, as everybody's life is a struggle. Tommy and Breda, congratulations to you, and thank you very much for having walked the walk and all the sacrifices you know best yourselves you've made for each other and your family. You fulfilled your promise, and God has blessed you hugely. This is the moment to rejoice and be thankful, and that's why we're here. We want to honour your life of commitment and blessings.

After the ceremony, we went to the Ardagh Hotel, where we had a beautiful night. The meal was delicious, the atmosphere was terrific, and all our family were there; I could not have asked for more. Sitting on the chair, I was so full of joy and pure delight that I couldn't help thinking, *This is what my wedding day was meant to be like.*

I've always looked back on our wedding day with deep sadness and regret. Now I have what happened in the church on our 50th wedding anniversary as one of the happiest memories of my life, an experience that completely overrides all that went before. What a remarkable, magnificent, incredible memory to have and treasure for the rest of my life.

Despite everything, I reached our golden wedding anniversary. Tommy and I are closer than ever. Life is good, and I have found my place of belonging in the world.

A LETTER TO PSYCHIATRY: A COMPLAINT AGAINST MY CARE

Whatever hope I had after surviving a cruel childhood and multiple harsh experiences up to the age of 22, when I went for help to the psychiatric services, you made things worse. You saw my symptoms, but you never saw me.

You failed me in failing to recognise that it was those horrific experiences that had a profound bearing on my state of health and not some chemical imbalance in my brain. You failed to listen deeply to the cry of my heart when I needed help to believe in my basic goodness.

At the root of my problems was the way I had been continuously physically assaulted as a child, and as a teenager I was sexually abused. But you never seemed to understand the impact of a life of trauma on my body, mind and relationships.

The one exception was when I was invited by the clinical director in St Vincent's Hospital's psychiatric unit, Dublin, to speak to a conference of doctors about what had reduced me to such an appalling state of health. I had no speech prepared. I was too unwell for that. I spoke from my heart. I finished by saying, 'I believe bad experiences of care can wreck a person's health just as much as any serious illness can.'

In late October 1995, I decided to take back control of my life. With my GP's help, I gradually weaned myself off the 15 tablets which I had been taking for the previous five years.

When I told the consultant psychiatrist that I was now off

all medication, he was so aggrieved by my decision he took away the only support I had. He gave orders to the support centre near my home not to allow me into the facility again unless I agreed to go back on Lithium.

There was no way I was going to do that. His coercive control left me distraught. Being denied the support I needed and depended on, I had nowhere to turn for help. My relationship with my husband became so strained that I ended up admitting to a priest, 'My marriage is falling apart at the seams.' He recommended a therapist, and I have never looked back since. Last year, Tommy and I celebrated our golden wedding anniversary.

Between 29 electric shock treatments and a bombardment of psychotropic drugs to my body, what breaks my heart most is that you undermined my ability to be a loving mother and wife. Your overly medical approach dimmed my mind to such an extent I no longer knew or trusted myself.

Your profession created untold damage to my life with its power and controlling behaviour towards me. The ECT treatments wiped out, completely and forever, all I had learned in university. All the classical music pieces that I could no longer play. You denied me the chance at a flourishing career. I could have been a great teacher. Instead, my health deteriorated to such an extent on your watch I no longer knew who I was. I was no longer able to make sense of my life or where it was going. My ability to be a loving wife and mother took such a severe hit and was so seriously undermined that it's a miracle my marriage survived.

My brain was fogged from the destructive impact of multiple psychotropic drugs. I drifted from moment to moment, hoping against hope that I'd make it through the day.

A LETTER TO PSYCHIATRY: A COMPLAINT AGAINST MY CARE

I find it incredible that I allowed psychiatry to have that kind of power over me, but it was as if my hands were tied. I was terrified of being prescribed even stronger drugs or hospitalised against my will. I have also been concerned about other people whose traumas have been ignored or left undetected. Were their families and the wider community denied the gift of their humanity? We all need to feel safe, heard, understood and valued.

Recently, my husband and I discussed what it was like for him over the 23 years I was under the care of various consultant psychiatrists. He said, 'You used to get upset over the smallest things. I was afraid to bring you anywhere. It was the frequency of the panic attacks. You were uncontrollable. It was outrageous. They could happen anywhere. As we were driving along, or in the house, wherever we were.'

I believe now that I was suffering from complex post-traumatic stress disorder (CPTSD). Unrecognised and unresolved traumas throughout my childhood and beyond were at the root of my bizarre behavioural reactions for years.

Tommy always said that the smallest thing used to upset me. Now I understand that people with CPTSD have low tolerance levels when it comes to words that are hurtful to them. When others would take no notice, CPTSD sufferers see it as an assault on their personhood. To this day, when I have a conversation with certain people, I'm on high alert in case something is said that I find hard to manage.

Since early adulthood, I've experienced how much ill-witted remarks can throw me. I believe now that I was suffering from complex PTSD as a result of not one but multiple traumas throughout my early years. I didn't know that was the reason that, without warning, my emotions flared up as they did. That's why I could not cope with overpowering emotions that erupted when least expected.

Learning about CPTSD has helped restore my self-respect. It has helped me to understand why some moderately upsetting event could become something I had to defend at all costs, as if my life depended on it. As if my character, my very essence as a person, was at stake. In my view, my distress was inappropriately labelled as a mental illness. I never suffered from bipolar disorder or manic depression, but I was hypersensitive and reacted poorly to any real or imagined threat from others.

I was not allowed to hold a different point of view or to have an active role in planning my recovery. Your oppressive hold on me intensified my agony instead of relieving it.

I'm still vulnerable. I still have my wounds and my scars. From time to time, I struggle with darkness in my life. I react poorly when someone says something hurtful or undermining. However, I also have developed skills to manage my emotions at those times. I have allowed other aspects of my personality to grow, meaning I now have other resources to draw on.

I have created a network of people around me in whose company I feel safe, respected and appreciated. I can turn to them in times of difficulty, and they will be there for me.

GLOSSARY OF MEDICATIONS AND TREATMENTS ADMINISTERED TO BREDA

Camcolit – A controlled-release lithium carbonate used in bipolar and recurrent depression.

ECT – Electroconvulsive therapy is a medical treatment most commonly used with severe major depression or bipolar disorder that has not responded to other treatments. Small electric currents pass through the brain, intentionally causing a brief seizure. The seizure is believed to alter brain chemistry.

Eltroxin – For treating thyroid hormone deficiency.

Faverin – An anti-depressant used to treat depression and obsessive-compulsive disorder (OCD).

Gamanil – An anti-depressant.

Gardenal – A barbiturate used to treat epilepsy. Barbiturates cause a decrease in brain activity. They may be used to treat insomnia, seizures and convulsions, and to relieve anxiety and tension before surgery.

Laroxyl – An anti-depressant.

Librium – From the Benzodiazepine family, a muscle relaxant that can become addictive over time.

Lithium – A mood stabiliser given to correct emotional dysregulation; commonly used when there is a diagnosis of bipolar. Requires monitoring as it can have serious side effects.

Melleril – An antipsychotic medication, it is a major tranquiliser used to treat psychosis.

Modecate – An anti-psychotic medication used to treat and control chronic schizophrenia and other mental illnesses.

Mogadon – A sedative prescribed for sleep difficulties.

Mysoline – A barbiturate used to treat epileptic seizures.

Nembutal – Another barbiturate that depresses the central nervous system. At low doses, it can help to initiate sleep, and at higher doses, it may may be used to treat severe anxiety.

Optimax – An anti-depressant for treatment-resistant depression.

Parnate/Parstelin – A potent anti-depressant given to patients who meet the criteria for major depression.

Prothiaden – An anti-depressant that can also reduce anxiety.

Psychotropic medication – A psychotropic describes any drug that affects behaviour, mood, thoughts, or perception. This can include medications for anxiety and depression as well as antipsychotics. These medications are believed to work by modifying levels of neurotransmitters in the brain.

Scoline – Used to cause short-term paralysis as part of general anaesthetic, given before ECT.

Seroxat – An anti-depressant, part of a modern group of medications known as SSRIs, believed to reduce depression by increasing the level of serotonin in the brain.

Sodium Amytal – Popularly known as the truth drug or truth serum, it is a barbiturate that is administered to help people to relax deeply. A hypnotic which is used for short-term treatment of insomnia, it is also an anaesthetic.

Surmontil – An anti-depressant which also has sedative effects and can be used to treat insomnia.

Valium – A tranquiliser that is highly addictive.

ACKNOWLEDGEMENTS

Writing a book turned out to be more complex than I initially imagined. Over the past four years, I have come to understand the extensive teamwork involved in creating such a work. This past year, in particular, has been eye-opening, expanding my perspective and allowing me to truly appreciate how much good can arise from challenging experiences when like-minded people work together.

I want to express my gratitude to clinical psychologist, Dr Tony Bates, whose unwavering support and belief in my story gave me the courage to embark on this writing journey after a failed attempt twenty-five years ago. His insightful feedback, constant encouragement and extraordinarily high standard of work on the manuscript motivated me through the most challenging times. I owe him a debt of gratitude.

I am deeply grateful to Gill for their pivotal role in bringing this book to fruition. Their support and dedication to the project have made my dream a reality. Sarah Liddy, who first interviewed me in Dublin, presented her team with the initial draft and oversaw the entire project. Charlie Lawlor, her colleague, worked closely with her and provided a powerful overview of the book for the cover, capturing its essence remarkably. Thank you both.

Liadán Hynes travelled from Dublin to the West of Ireland and spent a week with me here at home, interviewing me about different aspects of the book before she undertook the mammoth task of editing the story from a reader's point of view.

Subsequently, the manuscript was handed over to managing editor Margaret Farrelly, whose remarkable insights significantly enriched each chapter beyond my expectations. I was astonished when the contributions didn't end there. Sally Vince joined the effort, bringing a fresh perspective and meticulous attention to detail that greatly enhanced the clarity and impact of my narrative. To Liadán, Margaret and Sally, your dedication to quality and your belief in this project have been inspiring. Thank you for your part in making my dream come true.

I would also like to thank Kieran Kelly of Flynn O'Driscoll, Corporate Law Firm, for his painstaking work in providing a solicitor's report.

Looking back on my life, there are numerous others whose wisdom, love and expertise have been invaluable. I think of those who were signposts along the way and offered the help and support I urgently needed. No matter how small, each contribution, including yours, played a crucial role in my ability to keep going and, ultimately, in my recovery.

Sr Maura Hayes, who supported me when I was at my wit's end in the convent, and later her family, who allowed me to stay with them at weekends when I had nowhere else to go. Mary Sheehan, Catherine Delaney, Tomás Ó Canainn (in loving memory), Mrs Buckley, Mrs McCarthy, who befriended me when I was studying for a Bachelor of Music Degree in UCC. Health Nurse Mary Margaret Kyne, Dr Noel Walshe and the team in St Vincent's psychiatric unit, Elm Park, Dublin, November 1973. You gave me back a zest for life when I had none. You gave me hope.

Fr Austin Fergus, who was exceptionally good to me and

drove me back to St John of God psychiatric hospital in Dublin after a weekend at home, and stopped at Hayden's Hotel in Ballinasloe to buy me lunch. That day I couldn't get over his kindness and generosity. Fr Pat McGrath, Fr John Goode, Fr Paddy Tyrell, Fr John O'Gorman, Fr Raymond Flaherty and Canon James Ronayne, who has always had my best interests at heart and who supported this book from the start. Dr Brendan Flynn, founder of the Clifden Arts Festival in 1997 and its driving force ever since, who by his very presence in my life gave me courage during some of my darkest days.

Close friends Bernie and Willie Hughes; Margaret McDonagh of County Donegal; and Jacqueline Hannon, Nancy Duffy, and Gerry and Angela Coyne, who were the backbone of the adult choir and were always there for me. We had so much fun assisting with community events. Without realising it, each and every time we were together you gave me a renewed sense that life was worth living. Thank you.

Moreover, I will always cherish the excitement, delight and sense of accomplishment that primary school teacher Bernadette Conroy and I felt while working on a local nature booklet entitled 'Our Place', enriched with Bernadette's painstaking drawings and illustrations. We had an incredible time traveling from house to house, selling our 'masterpiece' to raise funds for a local charity. Bernadette, your mother and father Lily and Tom, held in loving memory, were always so warm and welcoming. I felt truly at peace and came home to myself in their presence. Thank you.

Similarly, I am grateful to Principal Mrs Marie Bourke, whose respect and high regard for my work as a music teacher always boosted my self-esteem and lifted my spirits. I also want to thank Eileen O'Malley and the other teachers in the school. Your zest for life and good humour energised and motivated me when no one knew how tough I was finding it to get through each day.

Regarding health and well-being, I owe a debt of gratitude to Fiona Brennan, Gerry and Miriam Hussey and the Soul Space Community, and Jason Quigley and the 'Rise and Thrive' members – 'The Mighty Ducks'. Vikki Grimes who founded 'Empower with Feel Good Fitness Workout Group', Peter Levine, Jane Negrych and the team in the Sanctuary founded by Sr Stan of Focus Ireland, Peter Dorai Raj, Dr Edith Eger, her grandson Jordan and the Soul Search Community. Kathleen Fitzgerald and all who helped me on the road to recovery. Last but not least Sr Marie Dunne CHF who travelled from Dublin to Connemara to be there and surprise us when the school choir under my direction performed her Mass in honour of St Brigid. Thank you Marie for your beautiful, uplifting and empowering friendship ever since.

I am also grateful to those no longer with us, whose loving care, kindness and friendship gifted me time and time again with a more positive outlook on life. Kitty Bence, my First Grade teacher. Dame Maura OSB and the Benedictine Sisters, and Wallie Murphy and Lena Goff, both highly regarded teachers in Kylemore Abbey who befriended me; Betty Fitzsimmons who ran Kylemore Post Office; Mary Ellen and Willie Aspell, who accepted me as one of their family; Agnes Nee; Mary Margaret O'Donnell, who was like an extraordinarily loving mother to me; Helen Cosgrove; and Kathleen and Tim Kelly. I will never forget your warmth and kindness that empowered me each day to keep going. Fr John McCarthy, Fr Michael Higgins and Fr Daniel O'Leary. Mrs Foyle, Clifden Bay Hotel, who gave me the opportunity of a lifetime when I needed it most. Each one of you gifted me with renewed strength, courage and hope. You believed in me when I didn't believe in myself.

I want to express my deepest gratitude to my family, whose unwavering encouragement and steadfast belief in me have been my guiding light. Your love and support have been my constant companions, and for that, I am eternally grateful. Your belief in my journey has been a source of endless strength and inspiration. Breda Ann, you told me that if I didn't write the book, you would! Suddenly, I realised, nobody knows the story as well as the one who has lived it. Your ultimatum gifted me with a determination and passion for the project that I didn't know I had.

To Tommy, for your incredible love, patience and forbearance, and for standing by me even through the most difficult years. Another man would have fled! My sincere apologies for all I put you through. Please forgive me.

To my five daughters, Fiona, Karen, Maria, Breda Ann and Marguerite. I deeply regret the hardships you faced during your childhood and formative years. Looking back, my greatest sorrow is that I wasn't a more loving mother who recognised the importance of nurturing your emotional needs alongside your physical ones. Please forgive my many faults, failings and weaknesses.

To my wonderful daughter's partner Derek, and sons-in-law, Jason, Joey and James. Though I lost three sons, I couldn't have been more blessed when each of you came as a wondrous gift into my life. Also, our extended family members, Leo (in fond remembrance) and Angela De Courcey; Peadar (in fond remembrance) and Winnie Ó Bríain; Cathy Coohill and family; Cyril Craughwell; and Lisa, Donald, Ellen and the rest of the Needham family. I could not ask for more wonderful, kind, generous, helpful and caring people in my life. I am surrounded by love.

Finally, to my beloved grandchildren, Michelle, Diarmuid, Finnán, Daithí, Conor, Leo, Daire, Aoife, Allie, Jake, Noah and Hannah. Thank you for filling my life with awe and wonder, as well as the love, joy, fun and laughter that had been missing for so long. I love you all, as Breda Ann said to me when she was young, and continues to do so, 'I love you to infinity and beyond.'